ENDOMETRIOSIS
Past, Present and Future

METHIL KANNAN KUTTY

MUHAMED T OSMAN

Copyright © 2018 Kannan Kutty & Osman

All rights reserved.

ISBN-13: 978-1720427694
ISBN-10: 1720427968

DEDICATION

This book is dedicated to all patients who have endometriosis.

Kannan Kutty and Osman

CONTENTS

	Foreword & Preface	i
1	Historical Background and Clinical Aspects of Endometriosis	9
2	Concept of Aetiopathogenesis of Endometriosis	35
3	Blood Biomarkers in Endometriosis	98
4	Imaging Endometriosis	118
5	Pharmacotherapy of Endometriosis	147
6	A Review of the Medical Treatment of Endometriosis	187
7	Psychosocial Manifestation of Endometriosis and Current Concept of management	204
8	Endometriosis and Future directions	217

FOREWORD

It is my honour to pen these few words for this erstwhile project to bring together a collection of writings on a disease that has troubled women for years – endometriosis. Who better to initiate this than my colleague, Professor Dr Kannan Kutty Methil, who needs no introduction to pathologists in Malaysia. He has many other characteristics worth emulating by persons starting out in the medical profession – determination, collegiality, knowledge, humility and curiosity among others. More enduring to me has been his friendship through the years.

Endometriosis is a great mimicker of illnesses in women. It is due to the formation of lesions and endometrium like tissues outside the uterus usually in the pelvic cavity. However, it can occur in many far flung areas like the deltoid muscle which often leads to diagnostic dilemmas. Endometriosis cases are more prevalent in infertile women (more than 8 times) compared to fertile women. It becomes a debilitating disease in such women, if not managed well, what more with the stress of not being able to conceive coupled with crippling pelvic pain.

In relevance to the causes, its pathogenesis is poorly understood yet some journals deduce certain risk factors and theories that may cause endometriosis. Genetics may play a role and increases the risk of endometriosis by 3-10 times. It is felt that genetics accounts for half the cases and the other half due to environmental/other factors. There has been growing interest in cellular and molecular alterations in the body's normal regulatory responses and pathway concerning core proteins and receptors. Several potential diagnostic markers have been associated with endometriosis. These markers such as Ca-125 have been used mainly in the management and diagnosis of late stage endometriosis. There has been increasing research interest in detecting markers for early stage disease as it has been found that laparoscopic treatment of the lesions during early stage disease doubles the rate of spontaneous pregnancy.

Laparoscopy has been the gold standard for diagnosis. An important chapter on imaging modalities discusses the use of the ultrasound, CT scan and the MRI in the diagnosis of endometriosis. The reader will get to know the false positives and false negatives of the various modalities in imaging. To be forewarned is to be forearmed!

Theories have abounded about the cause of endometriosis. According to the most common theory of ectopic endometrial cells (Sampson's theory of retrograde menstruation), endometrial cells flow backwards through the fallopian tubes and into the peritoneal cavity during menses. Other potential sources of ectopic endometrial cells include mesothelium, stem cells, Müllerian rests, bone marrow stem cells and embryonic vestiges as well as lymphatic or vascular dissemination and coelomic metaplasia. Evidence supporting retrograde menstruation comes from the observation that the incidence of endometriosis is increased in girls with genital tract obstructions that prevent drainage of menses through the vagina and therefore increase tubal reflux. However, while up to 90 percent of women have retrograde menstruation, most women do not develop endometriosis, which suggests that additional factors are involved.

Once endometriosis is established, the process appears to cause symptoms through inflammatory changes. Endometriosis-related pelvic pain is associated with increased production of inflammatory and pain mediators as well as neurologic dysfunction related to the implants. An increase of nerve fibresand imbalance of sympathetic and sensory nerve fibreshave been demonstrated in women with endometriosis-related pain. Proposed mechanisms for pain symptoms include oestrogen acting as a neuromodulator that selectively repulses the sympathetic axons while preserving sensory innervation, inflammation stimulating peripheral nerve sensitization, and chronic pain inducing changes in the central nervous system.

The mechanism for subfertility appears to involve anatomic distortion from pelvic adhesions and endometriomas and/or production of substances (e.g. prostanoids, cytokinesand growth factors) that are "hostile" to normal ovarian function/ovulation, fertilization, and implantation.

Medical treatment options include nonsteroidal analgesics, hormonal contraceptives, gonadotropin-releasing hormone (GnRH) agonists, and aromatase inhibitors. As there are no data supporting one treatment or treatment combination over another, the treatment choice is based upon symptom severity, patient preferences, medication side effects, treatment efficacy, contraceptive needs, costs, and availability.

Of note, medical interventions do not improve fertility, diminish endometriomas or treat complications of deep endometriosis such as ureteral obstruction. Women with these problems will need to proceed with therapy targeted at the specific problems.

Doctors should have exhaustive knowledge of the drugs that they use including being conversant with the side effects. There is a chapter devoted to the pharmacotherapy of endometriosis including newer drugs under clinical trial. Cost is an important consideration in the choice of these drugs. The practitioner is always advised to know any clinical practice guidelines that are locally applicable. These CPGs would indicate peer opinion on treatment options that may be offered to women.

All gynaecologists will realise that timing is critical in the choice of therapies, be it medical or surgical in the effective management of these patients. One can aim for pain relief with medication initially but once hormones are commenced in the management of endometriosis, one cannot continue this for a long duration without encountering side effects.

Similarly surgical interventions in women desirous of fertility should be timed correctly. Otherwise a women may be subjected to numerous surgeries during her reproductive life compromising her fertility with the formation of dense adhesions and tubal compromise. This clinical judgment will come with experience as well as knowledge gained from books such as this.

The inclusion of a chapter on psychosocial aspects of endometriosis is commendable. It recognises the tremendous burden on the mental health of a woman suffering from this chronic illness. As mentioned, there is a tendency to inadvertently underestimate the psychosocial management and its implication on the affected women. Attention has been drawn to issues at the workplace. Endometriosis is one of the important factors that affect women's productivity and self-esteem.

The reader will benefit from realising that women with this disease require a sympathetic ear to their symptoms. One should not dismiss the symptoms when there are no visible lesions on imaging. Often the smallest lesions are the most painful. The doctor must also be prepared for long term follow up of such patients. The family as well as the patient will need to be educated on the natural history of the disease and aims of treatment for the best results. This will carry the best outcome so that there is no undue pressure and expectation of unrealistic outcomes.

In my 35 years of experience in managing many women with endometriosis, the following has been my dictum which has always worked well for me.

A Avoid unrealistic targets
B Brief the patient fully at all steps
C Caring attitude
D Document well and stage the disease accurately
E Evidenced based therapy
F Frankness without raising unrealistic expectations.
G Guidance and being there for the patient.
H Holistic management

I am sure it will these dictums will serve you well as you manage cases of women with endometriosis.

Please enjoy the rest of the book. It is treasure trove of information on all aspects of endometriosis.

Professor Dato Dr Ravindran Jegasothy; FRCOG
Dean,
Faculty of Medicine,
MAHSA University,
Malaysia

PREFACE

The spectacle of amazing advances in the complex spectrum of the etiology, pathogenesis and treatment of gynecological disorders in general and endometriosis in particular provides an exciting venture for all those interested in current trends in gynecology and this is the raison d'etre for this book. Spectacular achievements in the state of the art technology and progressive discoveries such as microRNA etc has impacted all facets of medical disciplines in unraveling molecular mechanisms of diseases including endometriosis. Cognizant of this scenario adorned by the cutting edge of modern technology and its paramount importance in perceptive of the fundamentals of pathogenesis of endometriosis, a common disorder we have dealt with some of the breakthroughs for better comprehension of certain facets that have hitherto remained unclear. Endometriosis is a common gynecological disorder which is in fact a global menacing problem. Endometriosis affects more than 10 per cent of women in the reproductive years, with a peak incidence between the ages of 25 and 35. Although fairly common, it can be puzzling as the symptoms vary greatly in their type and severity. It is one of the commonest causes of pelvic pain and infertility in women worldwide. Commonly, several years may elapse before the diagnosis is made. Some women with sinister advanced disease have minimal pain but experience the sudden grief of discovering that they are infertile. It is also a cause of considerable morbidity and needless to reiterate its major impact on public health. We wish all the readers a salubrious journey through this book and if this book succeeds in providing the readers, be they doctors, postgraduate students, physicians or gynecologists, advantageous journey, we will feel a profound sense of satisfaction and achievement of our objectives of writing this. This book acknowledges appreciatively, sincerely and unreservedly all those responsible in one way or another, for stimulating us with their wisdom, experience and expertise.

Methil Kannan kutty; M.B.B.S., M.D., F.R.C.Path and F.R.C.P.A.

Muhamed T. Osman; M.B.Ch.B., M.Sc., Ph.D.

1 HISTORICAL BACKGROUND AND CLINICAL ASPECTS OF ENDOMETRIOSIS

Professor K. Siva Achanna; MBBS, FRCOG, FICS, FAMM

Dept. of Obstetrics & Gynaecology, Head of the Department, MAHSA University, Kuala Lumpur. Malaysia.

Introduction

Endometriosis is a benign disease defined by the presence of extrauterine endometrial stromal and glandular tissue. The disease discloses a broad spectrum of clinical signs and symptoms. Its pathophysiology is still not fully understood. Various theories exist including Sampson's well-known retrograde menstruation theory from the 1920s, which despite its imperfections still remains the most well-known. The three other pathophysiological theories are: coelomic metaplasia, haematogenous or lymphatic diffusion and immunological dysfunction. Coelomic metaplasia theory favours the existence of endometriotic lesions in premenarchal girls and distant sites. Both peritoneum and endometrium are derivatives of coelomic epithelium. Metaplasia is initiated from one coelomic-derived epithelium to the other [1]. Immunological dysfunction is the recent of hypotheses to explain disease progression and initiation.

The disease is susceptible to advancement and relapse. The pathogenesis and natural history of endometriosis remain implicit. However, with the introduction of modern molecular methods, new insights into the mechanisms of the disease, is yielding first-hand approaches to its diagnosis and treatment.

The cause is entirely ambiguous. Most often, the ovaries (common site), oviducts and tissue around the uterus back and front are affected [2]. The affected areas bleed each month, resulting in inflammation and scarring [3, 4]. Diagnosis is usually based on symptoms in combination with investigations including medical imaging (transvaginal ultrasonography, magnetic resonance imaging), tumour markers (CA-125) and histological evidence.

The mean age of diagnosis of endometriosis ranges between the thirties and forties and even as early as 8 years [5]. This condition is rare in premenarcheal girls. The overall prevalence of endometriosis in reproductive aged women probably is between 10% and 15% [6]. Early menarche and short menstrual cycles have been associated with increased risk of endometriosis [7]. Primate data have suggested exposure to environmental toxins-polychlorinated biphenyl (PCB) or dioxin linked to endometriosis, but produced inconsistent results [8].

Historical background of endometriosis

There has been a growing interest in the history of endometriosis. It has been documented in medical texts more than 4,000 years ago [9]. The Hippocratic Corpus illustrates symptoms similar to endometriosis, including uterine ulcers, adhesions and infertility [9]. Historically, women with these symptoms were treated with leeches, straitjackets, bloodletting, chemical douches, genital mutilation, pregnancy, hanging upside down, surgical intervention and even killing due to suspicion of demonic possession.

Nezhat et al. [10], made an exhaustive search in a number of classic texts from antiquity to the 19th century containing descriptions of symptoms which they compiled as proof of the actuality of endometriosis. Obviously, based on these symptoms of the condition, scholars disagree as to who was the first to establish the existence of endometriosis. The current definition of endometriosis therefore stands at the presence of functional endometrial-like tissue outside the uterus, but within the pelvic cavity or even outside with proof of cellular activity [11].

Previously, peritoneal, extraperitoneal, deep penetrating endometriosis, ovarian endometrioma (chocolate cysts) and adenomyosis (multi-faceted entities) were lumped together as "adenomyoma" until 1920s, did "adenomyoma" and endometriosis became separate diseases [12,13].

Ancient descriptions

In 1999, Knapp VJ, [14] listed a number of old dissertations dating back to from 17th to 18th centuries, acknowledged to the description of the features of endometriosis. However, in 2012, Nezhat *et al* [10], reiterated that even in ancient times, some of the writings have featured precisely the symptoms of endometriosis. In more recent times, such descriptions were confirmed with the histological findings of the presence of endometrial glands and stroma. On the other hand, the presence of symptoms such as pelvic pain, dysmenorrhoea, dyspareunia, and menorrhagia are unreliable symptoms to confirm a diagnosis of endometriosis.

Knapp VJ [14], has unearthed from the US National

library of Medicine many texts dealing with female health issues. Unfortunately, this material is abandoned by contemporary medical scholars. His work is primarily based on Schrön's *Disputatio inauguralis medica de ulceribus uteri,* which Knapp VJ considers "the first known and highly meticulous description of wide-ranging peritoneal endometriosis" [15]. There were however, many disagreements and difference of opinion on these issues.

Discovery of ovarian endometriosis

Carl Rokitansky, [16], perceived and labelled his cases as "sarcomas". Later Batt [17], interpreted Rokitansky utilizinga personal definition of tumours, the opus magnum (A Manual of Pathological Anatomy) [18]. Emge [19], analyzing Rokitansky's work formed the impression that his usage of the term "sarcoma" was meant to indicate an abnormally active proliferation of stroma rather than a truly malignant process.

Under the microscope, Russel [20] found a number of areas, which were exact prototype of the uterine glands and interglandular connective tissue and he believed the tumour was due to the presence of aberrant portions of müllerian duct in the ovary. In the renowned 1921 publication "Perforating haemorrhagic cysts of the ovary" [21], Sampson described 23 cases of ovarian haematomas of endometrial types varying from 1 to 9 cm in diameter. At operation the cyst or ovary was found to be adherent and whilst releasing it, "chocolate-like" material oozed out. Adhesions were seen in all cases, varying in location and the extent. In 1922, Sampson described a series of 37 cases of superficial and deep "chocolate cysts". At this stage, Sampson opined the ovary as an incubator, or intermediary horde in the development of pelvic implantation of adenomas of endometrial type. Later Sampson [22], assumed that rupture of the endometrial cyst was the cause of peritoneal endometriosis. Halban's [23] explanation of the lymphatic theory, Brosens *et al* [24] demonstration of muscle metaplasia, is of enormous importance in the understanding the pathophysiology and proper management of endometrioma.

The documentation of adenomyoma

In the general description of Rokitansky's autopsy findings [25], he alludes to some "rare cases where there is extension of the uterine glands occurred in both directions, i.e. both into the uterus cavity and the uterus parenchyma. Search of literature identified 13 reports of "adenomyomatus polyps") mostly by Japanese authors, structures that resemble endometrial polyps containing a smooth muscle component.

The name adenomyoma was devised towards the end of 19th century. In 1896, Cullen and Von Recklinghausen described the condition [26, 27]. Subsequently in 1897 Pick [28] and Rolly [29, 30], contributed to this. Twenty years later, Lockyer [31] provided a comprehensive definition. The term "adenomyoma" denotes a new formation composed of gland-elements, hyperplastic cellular connective tissue and smooth muscle.

Cullen [12] collected 90 uteri with adenomyomas and described their various presentations. His specimens were from the myometrial wall, uterine horns, the subserosa, uterine ligaments and ovaries. Here he appreciated the continuity between eutopic endometrial glands and the nests in the myometrium. Also Cullen considered uterine adenomyoma, ovarian endometriosis and deep endometriosis as one disease culminating by the presence of endometrial tissue outside the uterine mucosa.

Clinical aspects of endometriosis

Endometriosis is a disease with considerable

prevalence. The disease has several impacts in general, physical, mental and social well-being. Diagnostic delay of endometriosis is a problematic issue [32] and it takes 8 to 10 years to be diagnosed with long, expensive diagnostic tools [33,34].Common elements in the history include nulliparity, irregular menstrual cycles, pain usually precedes flow by a few days and begins to resolve in 1-2 days into the menses.

The main symptoms are pelvic pain and subfertility. Pain also occurs at the time of sexual intercourse. Subfertility occurs in up to half of women affected [3].A familial/genetic predisposition has been documented. A woman with a first-degree relative with endometriosis has a lifetime risk of the disease approximately 10 times that of a woman without as affected family member. Symptoms of endometriosis can be inconstant but characteristically mirror the anatomical area of involvement. Such symptoms may include the following:

- Dysmenorrhoea
- Heavy or irregular periods
- Chronic Pelvic pain
- Lower abdominal or back pain
- Deep dyspareunia
- Dyschezia
- Feeling of bloating, nausea and vomiting
- Inguinal pan
- Pain on micturition
- Pain during exercise

The cyclical proliferation, shedding and bleeding of the ectopic endometrium results in inflammation, adhesions, scarring and seemingly, chronic pelvic pain[35]or adnexal masses[36].Sexual dysfunction is also more common in women with advanced-stage endometriosis secondary to dyspareunia [37] from deep deposits of disease within the uterosacral ligaments or rectovaginal septum.[Fig. 1]

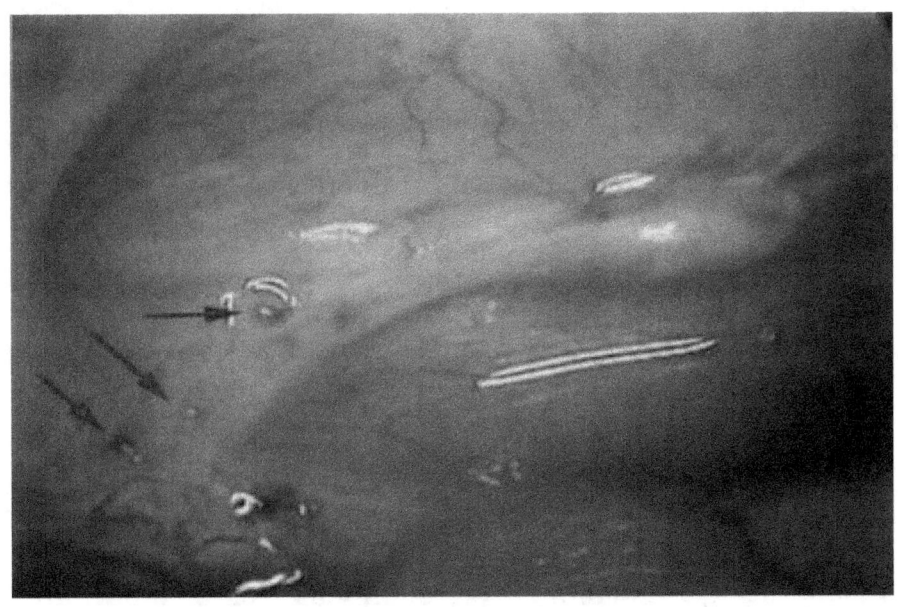

Figure 1. Appearance of Minimal Endometriosis on the Uterosacral ligaments

Physical Examination

In general, patients with endometriosis do not have any specific clinical findings apart from non-specific tenderness at the sites of the disease. Pelvic examination may reveal exaggerated tenderness particularly during menstruation. The hallmark of the findings is usually nodular thickenings along the uterosacral ligaments, obliteration and distortion of the pelvic anatomy and fixed retroversion of the uterus. At times, bluish nodules maybe seen in the vagina due to infiltration from the posterior vaginal wall. Rupture of an endometrioma may present as a case of acute abdomen.

Widespread involvement of the rectum and other sites of the gastro intestinal tract may cause extensive adhesion formation leading to intestinal obstruction, pain, tenderness and surgical guarding. Excessive endometrial angiogenesis has been suggested as a mechanism in the pathogenesis of endometriosis. The ectopic endometrium of women with this disorder has an increased capacity to proliferate, implant and grow in the peritoneum [38]. Endometrium is a rich source of growth factors that promote angiogenesis, including fibroblast growth factors and vascular endometrial growth factor [39, 40, and 41]. Interleukin-8 is a chemoattractant and activating factor for human neutrophils and a potent angiogenic agent. Interleukin-8, prostanoids, macrophages and cytokine concentrations in peritoneal fluid show higher levels among women with endometriosis, according to the stage of the disease, when compared with controls. Peritoneal fluid of women with endometriosis has been shown to have a direct toxic effect on both sperm and embryos in vitro [42, 43]It has been also suggested exposure to environmental pollutants, especially dioxin (a toxic substance formed by incenerating chlorine based chemical waste containing hydrocarbons), plays a role in causing endometriosis [8, 44].

Differential Diagnosis

- Ectopic pregnancy
- Pelvic inflammatory disease
- Diverticulitis
- Torsion of an ovary
- Appendicitis
- Bowel obstruction
- Pelvic adhesions
- Functional or neoplastic ovarian cyst
- Urinary tract infection

Combination of pelvic examination and pelvic ultrasonography in the form of transvaginal or endorectal are inexpensive, widely available and affordable particularly when used by experienced operators. The features vary from simple cysts to complex cysts with internal echos, devoid of vascularity. Other imaging techniques are computed tomography (CT) scanning, and magnetic resonance imaging (MRI). The latter is however expensive, less accessible and cannot conclusively be used to exclude endometriosis. It is the responsibility of the patient to disclose any possibility of pregnancy. Structured approach to counsel pregnant women about diagnostic imaging is pivotal.

Laparoscopy is used more frequently as a diagnostic tool. Diagnostic laparoscopy facilitates surgical visual inspection of the pelvic organs by an experienced surgeon.

Intravenous pyelography and colon studies maybe indicated when extra genital involvement is suspected. Hysterosalpingography may disclose occlusion of the oviducts or peri-adnexal adhesions.

Laboratory studies

A complete Full blood count inclusive of haemoglobin level to assess the level of blood loss with differential count may help to differentiate pelvic infection from endometriosis. Urinalysis and culture is mandatory if urinary tract infection is suspected.

Cervical gram stain and culture is also considered to rule out sexually transmitted diseases which can give rise to pelvic pain and subfertility. Serum markers do not provide adequate diagnostic accuracy. In some centres, serum cancer antigen 125 (CA-125) test is performed and is valid in advanced stage of the disease. The results are useful to measure the treatment response. CA-125 is a cell surface antigen expressed by derivatives of coelomic epithelium and is a well-established marker for monitoring of women with epithelial ovarian cancer. On the whole, the serum CA-125 concentration does not possess sufficient sensitivity to be considered a potent screening test for the diagnosis of endometriosis.

The preferred method of diagnosis is surgical visual inspection and examination of the excised material as the gold standard for the diagnosis of endometriosis. This requires the services of a skilled and experienced surgeon. The classic peritoneal implant is a blue-black "powder burn "lesions containing haemosiderin deposits from entrapped blood. [Fig. 2].

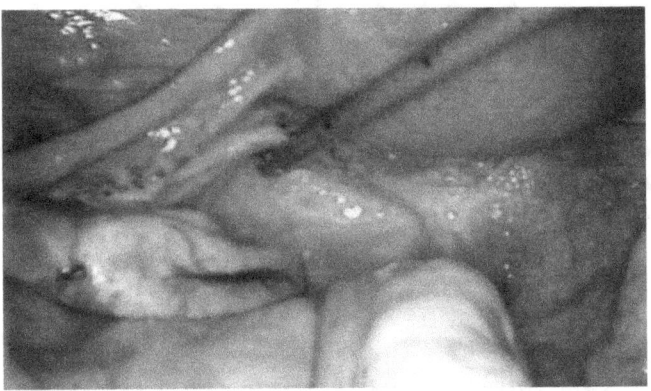

Figure 2. Powder-Burn lesion of endometriosis

Symptoms of endometriosis:

Dysmenorrhoea

Dysmenorrhoea is a common condition of women in their reproductive years. The term dysmenorrhea is derived from the Greek words *dys*, meaning difficult/painful; *meno*, month and *rrhea*, to flow. Local factors and centralized response to pain are thought to be involved in the pathophysiology. The majority of women will respond to medical treatments. The role of surgical treatment is rather small. More evidence is now available on the use of complementary therapies to treat dysmenorrhea.

Primary dysmenorrhea appears multifactorial. This entity typically presents 6-12 months after menarche. Pain is cramping in nature, occurs in the lower abdomen and may radiate to the back or thighs. Towards the end of menstrual cycle, progesterone decline triggers various inflammatory cytokines, prostaglandins, vascular endothelial growth factors (VEGFs) and several matrix metalloproteinases (MMPs), leading to loss of integrity of blood vessels, destruction of endometrial interstitial matrix.

The uterine contraction and vasoconstriction theory presently has a strong scientific basis of pain. Other factors involved in the sensation of pain include leukotrienes, vasopressin and a reduction in prostacyclin levels. Leukotrienes increase myometrial contraction and vasoconstriction. Women who fail to respond to prostaglandin inhibitors have been shown to have elevated levels of leukotrienes [45].

Secondary dysmenorrhea is as a result of pelvic pathology. Usually occurs a number of years after menarche and pain may occur throughout the secretory phase of the menstrual cycle as well as the menstruation. The most common cause of secondary dysmenorrhea is endometriosis. The exact mechanism as to how ectopic endometrial tissue causes pain is not precisely endorsed. Some studies have established increased levels of prostaglandin F2α [46]. Another common cause of secondary dysmenorrhea is pelvic inflammatory disease. The pain is related to release of inflammatory mediators, prostaglandins, scar tissue formation and uterine contractions. Physical examination, maybe normal in primary dysmenorrhea, whilst findings maybe abnormal in secondary dysmenorrhea, depending on the underlying pathology.

Chronic pelvic pain

Chronic pelvic pain is a common condition in women of reproductive age group. It occurs in 14-24% of women aged between 18-50 years [47, 48]. Diagnostic laparoscopic findings in women who suffer from this melody, adhesions contribute to 24%, endometriosis 33% and no pathology in 35% of patients. Adhesions or endometriosis my not associate with the site or severity of pain. This discrepancy could be due to a complex neurophysiology of visceral sensation, particularly arising from the uterus and ovaries.

Pain is the most common symptom of endometriosis. The mechanisms involved largely remains unknown. Pain sensation is itself is difficult to define particularly if it is chronic. Chronic pelvic pain has a tendency to involve surrounding organ systems. Besides, the perception andtoleranceof pain varies with the individual. Tender nodularity in the cul-de-sac and along the uterosacral ligaments may contribute to dyspareunia and low back pain. When combined with laparoscopic ablation, significantly reduces pain attributed to endometriosis [49] and increased cumulative pregnancy rates [50]. Approach to the treatment of chronic pelvic pain is better dealt by multidisciplinary strategies. The team consists of a clinical psychologist, a physician with special interest in pain management and a gynaecologist. The limitation to this concept is the cost involved and recruiting manpower with passion for this job. Whilst hormone therapy controls ovarian activity, psychological approaches increase coping skills and reduce pain associated distress.

Medical treatment that involves inhibition of ovulation had been found to be effective in reducing pain in 80-90% of women [51]. Medical therapy is not cytoreductive, hence recurrence is frequent once the drug is withdrawn. [52].Furthermore, side effects and costs prohibit long term use and do not improve pregnancy rates in women presenting with subfertility.

Of late, technological advances in camera optics, electrosurgical devices and improved surgical skills, now make operative laparoscopy a favoured modality of treatment. Endometriotic implants can be seen throughout the pelvic peritoneum. Laparoscopic ablation using a carbon dioxide (CO_2) laser was first introduced in the early 1980s [Fig. 3].

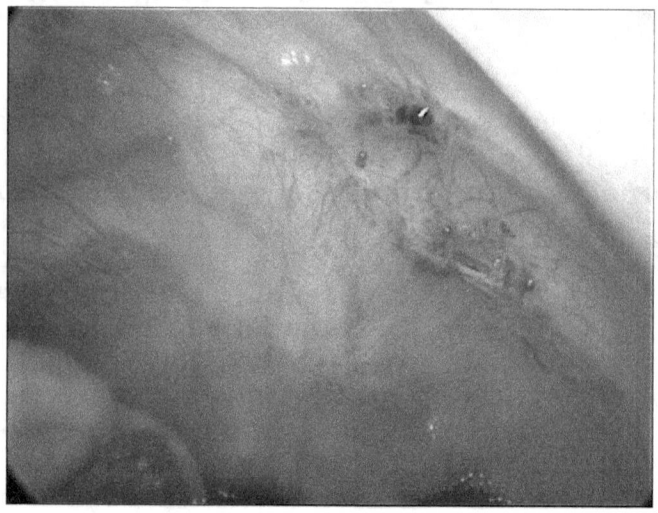

Figure 3: Laproscopic image of endometriotic lesions at the peritoneum of the pelvic wall

Since then, more new modalities for ablation have emerged: bipolar diathermy, monopolar electrosurgery, bipolar scissors and the harmonic scalpel. According to current available evidence, only 62.5% of women improve following laparoscopic ablation [53]. This could be due to deeper infiltrative disease. The latter patients were found to benefit from excisional surgery, which requires higher level of training. [Fig. 4].

Pelvic denervation can be used to interrupt the sensory nerve supply to the uterus in an attempt to reduce symptoms of dysmenorrhea. The commonly described procedure is laparoscopic uterine nerve ablation (LUNA) and presacral neurectomy (PSN), which are performed to interrupt the pain fibres. LUNA involves dividing the sensory parasympathetic fibres to the cervix and the sensory sympathetic fibres to the uterus contained in the cervical division of the Lee-

Frankenhauser plexus using a CO2 laser or electrosurgery. Potential complications of this procedure include uterine prolapse and pelvic denervation. The results of Vercellini *et al* [54] showed no difference in the perception of menstrual pain in one year one year after surgery, with 75% in the LUNA group and 74% in the excisional surgery group.

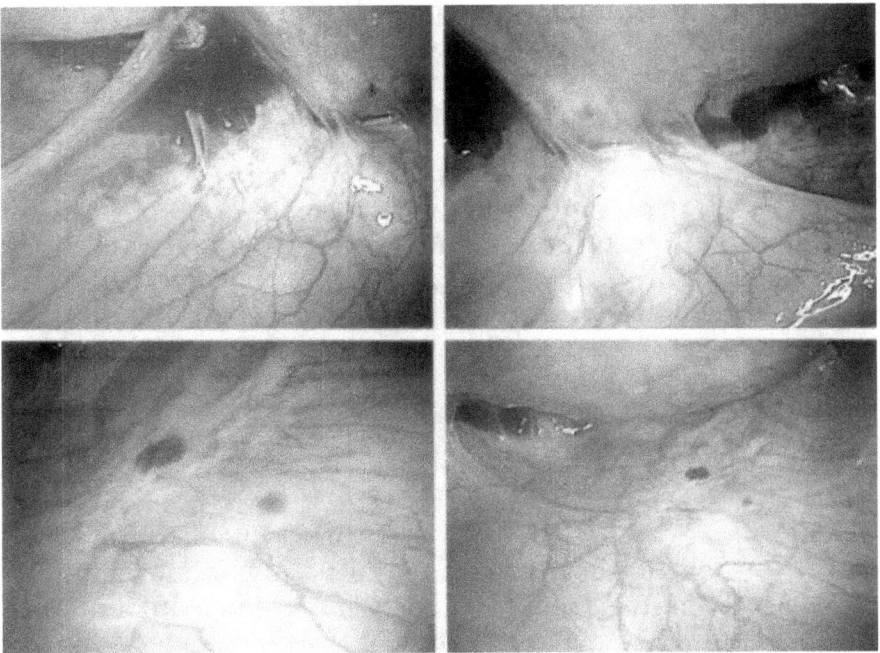

Figure 4. Active Endometriosis with red and powder-burn lesions and adhesion from old scarring

Adenomyosis

The first description of the condition were made by Karl von Rokitansky in 1860 [55], and von Recklinghausen in 1896 [56]. Adenomyosis uteri is defined by the presence of endometrium within the myometrium. There is no consensus in the depth of endometrial penetration diagnostic of adenomyosis uteri.

A cut-off point of >2.5mm for glandular extension below the endometrial-myometrial interface is supported [57]. Adenomyosis uteri can involve the whole muscle thickness till the serosa which can be "focal" or "diffuse". In the latter type, the uterus becomes enlarged and globular.

Associated Pathology; About 80% of women with adenomyosis also have other lesions, most frequent being leiomyomas. Endometrial polyps, hyperplasia with or without atypia and adenocarcinoma are frequent in women with adenomyosis uteri. Pelvic endometriosis is observed in 6-24% of women.

Adenomyosis uteriis also known to result from abnormal growth and invagination of the basal endometrium into the subendometrial myometrium at the endometrial-myometrial interface. Local but not systemic, hyperestrogen state may also account for hypertrophy/hyperplasiain the surrounding myometrium and overlying endometrium.

Clinical Correlates

As much as 35% of women with adenomyosis are asymptomatic whereas (40-50%) present with menstrual disorders in the form of menorrhagia, dysmenorrhea (10-30%)and metrorrhagia (10-12%), and infrequently dyspareunia or dyschesia [58,59].

Endometriosis. Pelvic endometriosis co-exists with adenomyosis in 2-24% of patients. Kunz et al[60], hypothesize that pelvic endometriosis and uterine adenomyosis are variants of the same disease, involving dislocation of the basal endometrium and the peritoneal cavity.

Adenomyosis uteri remain one of the most common pathological findings in hysterectomy specimens. Therefore, aiming for better diagnosis and specific therapy to reduce hysterectomy rates is of paramount importance. With better imaging modalities, accurate diagnosis is becoming better. Preoperative diagnosis facilitates more specific therapy and can be useful for counselling for non-invasive procedures.

Endometriosis and subfertility

Peritubal and periovarian adhesions can interfere mechanically with ovum transport leading to subfertility. Peritoneal endometriosis has been claimed to contribute to subfertility by interfering with tubal motility, folliculogenesis and corpus luteum function. Endometriosis may also cause subfertility by causing more sperm binding to the ampullary epithelium, thereby sperm-endosalpingeal interactions [61]. Medical treatment for minimal to mild has not been seen to increase pregnancy rates [62]. Moderate to severe have yielded better pregnancy rates with surgery [63]. Other choices for achieving pregnancy include: intrauterine insemination, superovulation and in vitro fertilization. In a case-controlled study, pregnancy success by intracytoplasmic sperm injection was not related to the presence or extent of endometriosis [64].

Some experts believe that endometriosis should be suppressed prophylactically with the usage of continuous ovulation inhibition drugs such as combined contraceptive pill, GnRH analogs, medroxyprogesterone acetate or danazol. These agents will cause regression of asymptomatic disease and would improve subsequent pregnancy rates. However, the Cochrane review refutes this opinion [65]. Surgical ablation of asymptomatic endometriosis has shown improvement of fecundity rates and enhance pregnancy rates [63]. In a systemic review, aromatase inhibitors were shown to have promising results with pain relief when combined with progestins, combined contraceptive pills or GnRH analogues. The GnRH analogues produce a hypogonadotrophic-hypogonadic state by down regulation of the pituitary gland.

Conclusion

Endometriosis was documented in medical text books more than 4,000 years ago, but first discovered by Karl von Rokitansky in 1860. Clinical diagnosis of pelvic endometriosis is a difficult task. Therefore, significant amounts of efforts are needed to improve the clinical diagnosis. Diagnostic considerations including skilled history taking, physical examination, laboratory studies and imaging techniques are invaluable. In addition, laparoscopic examination by experienced reproductive surgeons is the key to diagnosis and staging the extent of the disease.

Established medical therapies for the treatment of pain associated with endometriosis include estrogen-progestin contraceptives, progestins, GnRH agonists and danazol. No one medical treatment is ideal considering pain relief and recurrence rates. Treatment decisions must be individualized based on severity of symptoms, the extent of the disease, desire for pregnancy, age of the patients, side effects and costs. Aromatase inhibitors are another promising therapeutic option. On the whole, there is no significant evidence that medical treatment of endometriosis improves fertility.

The objectives of surgical treatments for endometriosis are to refurbish normal anatomical architecture and to excise all visible disease and prevent recurrence. Laparoscopy offers better visualization of the disease, less tissue trauma and desiccation, smaller incisions, speedy post-operative recovery and short hospital stay.

References

[1] Matsuura K, Ohtake H, KatabuchiH, Okamura H. Coelomic metaplasia theory of endometriosis: evidence from in vivo studies and an in vitro experimental model. Gynecol Obstet Invest 1999; 47 Suppl 1:18-20.

[2] "Endometriosis". http://www.womens health.gov/. December 5, 2014. Retrieved 4 March 2015. External link in/ website.

[3] Bulletti C, Coccia ME, Battisoni S, Borini A. "Endometriosis and Infertility". J Assist. Reprod. Genet. 2010; 27(8): 441-7.

[4] "Endometriosis overview". http://www.nichd.nih.gov.2013-06-24. Retrieved 4 March 2015.

[5] Vercellini P, Eskenazi B, Consonni D, Somigliana E, Parazzini F, Abbiati A, Fidele L. "Oral contraceptives and

risk of endometriosis: a systemic review and meta-analysis. Hum Reprod Update 2011; 17 (2): 159-70.

[6] Yi KW, Shin JH, Park MS, Kim T, Kim SH, Hur JY. Association of body mass index with severity of endometriosis in Korean women. Int J Gynaecol Obstet. 2009; 105: 39-42.

[7] Treloar SA, Bell TA, Nagle CM, Purdie DM, Green AC. Early menstrual charecteristics associated with subsequent diagnosis of endometriosis. Am J Obstet Gynecol. 2010; 202: 534-6.

[8] Guo SW, Simsa P, Kyama CM, et al. "Reassuring the evidence for the link between dioxin and endometriosis: from molecular biology to clinical epidemiology". Molecullar Human Reproduction 2009; 15 (10): 609-24.

[9] Nezhat C, Nezhat F. "Endometriosis: ancient disease, ancient treatments". Fertility & Sterility 2012; 98 (6 Suppl): S1-62..

[10] Nezhat C, Nezhat F. "Endometriosis: ancient disease, ancient treatments". Fertility & Steril 2012; 98 (6 Suppl): S1-62.

[11] Benagiano G, Brosens I: Who identified endometriosis? Fertil Steril 2011; 95: 13-16.

[12] Cullen TS, The distribution of adenomyomata containing uterine mucosa. Arch Surg 1920; 1: 215-283.

[13] Frankl O, Adenomyosis uteri. Am j Obstet Gynecol 1925; 10: 680-684.

[14] Knapp VJ: How old is endometriosis? Late 17th and 18th-century European descriptions of the disease. Fertil Steril 1999; 72: 10-14.

[15] Schrön D: Disputatio inauguralis medica de ulceribus uteri. Jena. Rudolf Wilhem Crause, Literis Krebsianis, 1690, pp 6-17.

[16] Benagiano G, Brosens I: The history of

endometriosis: identifying the disease. Hum Reprod 1991; 6: 963-968.

[17] Batt RE: A history of Endometriosis. London, Springer, 2011.

[18] Rokitansky C: A manual of Pathological Anatomy (transl by W.E. Swaine). Philadelphia, Blanchard & Lea, 1855, vol ¡: General pathological anatomy, pp 189-190.

[19] Emge LA: The elusive adenomyosis of the uterus. Its historical past and its present state of recognition. Am J Obstet Gynecol 1962; 83: 1541-1563.

[20] Russel WW: Aberrant portions of the müllerian duct found in an ovary. Johns Hopkins Hospital Bull 1899; 10: 8-10.

[21] Sampson JA: Perforating hemorrhagic (chocolate) cysts of the ovary. Arch Surg 1921; 3: 245-323.

[22] Sampson JA: Peritoneal endometriosis due to the menstrual dissemination of the endometrial tissue into the peritoneal cavity. Am J Obstet Gynecol 1927; 14: 422-469.

[23] Halban J: Hysteroadenosis metastatica. Die lymphogene Genese der sog. Adenofibromatosis heterotopic(Metastatic hysteroadenosis. The lymphatic origin of the so-called heterotopic adenofibromatosis). Arch Gynakol 1925; 124: 457-482.

[24] Brosens IA, Puttemans PJ, Deprest J: The endoscopic localization of endometrial implants in the ovarian chocolate cyst. Fertil Steril 1994; 61:1034-1038.

[25] Rokitansky C: Uber Uterusdrüsen-Neubildung in Uterus-und Ovarial-Sarcomen. (On the neoplasm of uterus glands on uterine and ovarian sarcomas). Zeitschr Ges Aerzte Wien 1860; 16: 577-581.

[26] Cullen T: Adenomyoma of the round ligament. Johns Hopkins Hosp Bull 1896;7: 112-113.

[27] Von Recklinghausen F: Die Adenomyomata und Cystadenomata der Uterus-und Tubenwandund: ihre Abkunft von Resten des Wolffischen KÖrpers (The Adenomyomas and Cystadenomas of the Uterus and Tube Wall: Their Origin from Remnants of the Wolffian Body). Berlin, Hirschwald, 1896.

[28] Pick L:Ein neuer Typus des voluminÖsen paroophoralen Adenomyomas-zugleich über eine bisher nicht bekannte Geschwulstform der Gebarmutter (Adenomyoma psammopapillare) und über totale Verdoppelung des Eileiters (A new type of voluminous paroophoral adenomyomas – both on a previously unknown form of the uterus (adenomyoma psammapapillare) and a total doubling of the oviduct). Arch Gynakol 1897; 54:117-206.

[29] Rolly F: Ueber einen Fall von Adenomyoma uteri mit Uebergang in Carcinom und Metastasenbildung (About a case of uterine adenomyoma with transition to carcinoma and metastasis). Arch Pathol Anat Physiol Klin Med 1897; 150: 555-582.

[30] Rolly F: Ueber einen Fall von Adenomyoma uteri etc. (About a case of adenomyoma of the uterus etc.). Virchows Arch 1897; 150:555.

[31] Lockyer C: Fibroids and Allied Tumours (Myoma and Adenomyoma). London, MacMillan, 1918.

[32] Hudelist G, Fritzer N, Thomas A, niehues C, Oppelt P, Haas D, et al. Diagnostic delay for endometriosis in Austria and Germany: causes and possible consequences. Hum Reprod. 2012; 27:3412-6.

[33] Luisi S, Lazzeri L, Ciani V, Petraglia F. Endometriosis in Italy: from cost estimates to new medical treatment. Gynecol Endocrinol. 2009; 25: 734-40.

[34] Rogers PA, D'Hooghe TM, Fazleabas A, Gargett CE, Giudice LC, Montgomery GW, et al. Priorities for endometriosis research : recommendations from an international consensus workshop. Reprod Sci. 2009; 16:

335-46.

[35] Bloski T, Pierson R. Endometriosis and chronic pelvic pain: unraveling the mystery behind this complex condition. Nurs Womens Health 2008; 12: 382-95.

[36] Practice Committee of the American Society for Reproductive Medicine. Endometriosis and Infertility: a committee opinion. Fertil Steril 2012; 98: 591-8.

[37] Garry R, Clayton R, Hawe J. The effect of endometriosis and its radical laparoscopic excision on quality of life indicators. Br J Obstet Gynaecol 2000; 107: 44-54.

[38] Hii LL, Rogers PA. Endometrial vascular and glandular expression of integrin alpha (v)beta3 in women with and without endometriosis. Hum Reprod 1998; 13:1030-5.

[39] Ferriani RA, Charnock-Jones DS, Prentice A, Thomas EJ, Smith SK. Immunohistochemical localization of acidic and basic fibroblast growth factor in normal human endometrium and endometriosis and the detection of their mRNA by polymerase chain reaction. Hum Reprod 1993; 8: 11-6.

[40] Charnock-Jones DS, Sharkey AM, Rajput-Williams J, Burch D, Schofield JP, Fountain SA, et al. Identification and localization of alternately spliced mRNAs for vascular endothelial growth factor in human uterus and steroid regulation in endometrial carcinoma cell lines. Biol Reprod 1993; 48:1120-8.

[41] Sangha K, XiaoFeng L, Shams M, Ahmed A. Fibroblast growth factor receptor-1 is a critical component for endometrial remodeling. Lab Invest 1997; 77: 389-402.

[42] Morcos RN, Gibbons WE, Findley We. Effect of peritoneal fluid on in vitro cleavage of 2-cell mouse embryos: possible role in infertility associated endometriosis. Fertil Steril 1985; 44: 678-83.

[43] Halme J, Hall JL. Effect of pelvic fluid from endometriosis patients on human sperm penetration of zona- free hamster ova. Fertil Steril 1982; 37: 573-6.

[44] Rier SE, Martin DC, Bowman RE, Dmowski WP, Becker JL. Endometriosis in rhesus monkeys (Macaca mullata) following chronic exposure to 2,3,7,8 tetraachlorodibenzo-p-dioxin. Fundam Appl Toxicol 1993; 21: 433-41.

[45] Demers LM, Hahn DW, McGuire JL. Newer concepts in dysmenorrhea research: leukotrienes and calcium channel blockers. In: Dawood MY, McGuire JL, Demers LM, editors. Premenstrual Syndrome and Dysmenorrhea. Baltimore: Urban & Schwarzenberg; 1985.p.205.

[46] Koike H, Ikenoue T, Mori N. (Studies on prostaglandin production relating to the mechanism of dysmenorrhea in endometriosis). Nippon Naibunpi Gakkai Zasshi 1994; 70:43-56.

[47] Mathias SD, Kuppermann M, Liberman RF, Lipschutz RC, Steege RF. Chronic pelvic pain: prevalence, health related quality of life, and economic correlates. Obstet Gynecol 1996; 87:321-7.

[48] Zondervan KT, Yudkin PL, Vessey MP, Jenkinson CP, Dawes MG, Barlow DH, et al. The community prevalence of chronic pelvic pain in women with associated illness behavior. Br J Gen Pract 2001; 51:541-7.

[49] Strattan P, Berkley KJ. Chronic pelvic pain and endometriosis: translational evidence of relationship and implications. Hum. Reprod. Update. 2011, 17 (3): 327-46.

[50] "Diagnosis and Treatment of Endometriosis". American Academy of Family Physcicians. 1999-10-15. Retrieved 2011-07-26.

[51] Prentice A, Deary AJ, Goldbeck-Wood S, Farquhar C, Smith SK. Gonadotrophin-releasing hormone analogues for pain associated with endometriosis. Cochrane Database Syst Rev 2000; 2: CD000346.

[52] Miller JD, Shaw RW, Casper RF, Rock JA, Thomas EJ, Dmowski WP, et al. Historical prospective cohort study of the recurrence of pain after discontinuation of treatment with danazol or a gonadotropin-releasing hormone agonist. Fertil Steril 1998; 70: 293-6.

[53] Sutton CJ, Ewen SP, Whitelaw N. Haines P. Prospective, randomized, double blind, controlled trial of laser laparoscopy in the treatment of pelvic pain asoociated with minimal, and moderate endometriosis. Fertil Steril 1994; 62: 696-700.

[54] Vercellini P, Aimi G, Busacca M, Apolone G, Uglietti A, Crosignani PG. Laparoscopic uterosacral ligament resection for dysmenorrhea associated with endometriosis: results of a randomized, controlled trial. Fertil Steril 2003; 80:310-9.

[55] Von Rokitansky C. Ueber uterusdrusen- nebildung in uterus-und ovarial-sarcomen. (Article in German) Ztsch K K Gesellsch der Aerzte zu Wien 1860; 37: 577-81.

[56] Von Recklinghausen F. Die Adenomyomata und Cystadenomata der Uterus und Tubenwandung: Ihre Abkunft von Resten des Wolff'schen Koerpes. (Article in German). Berlin: August Hirschwald Verlag; 1896.

[57] Uduwela AS, Perera MA, Aiqing L, Fraser IS. Endometrial-myometrial interphase relationship to adenomyosis and changes in pregnancy. Obstet Gynecol Surv 2000: 390-400.

[58] Parazzini F, Vercellini P, Panazza S, Chatenhoud L, Oldani S, CrosignaniPG. Risk factors for adenomyosis. Hum Reprod 1997: 1275-9.

[59] Vavillis D, Agorastos T, Tzafetas J, Loufopoulos A, Vakiani, Constantinidis T. et al. Adenomyosis at hysterectomy: prevalence and relationship to operative findings and reproductive and menstrual factors. Clin Exp Obstet Gynecol 1997; 24:36-8.

[60] Kunz G, Bell D, Huppert P, Leyendecker G,.

Structural abnormalities of the uterine wall I women with endometriosis and infertility visualized by sonography and magnetic resonance imaging. Human Reprod 2000; 15: 76-82.

[61] Reeve L, Lashen H, Pacey AA, Endometriosis affects sperm endo-salpingeal interactions. Hum Reprod 2005; 20(2): 448-51.

[62] Badawy SZ, Elbakry MM, Samuel F, Diger M. Cumulative pregnancy rates in infertile women with endometriosis. J Reprod Med 1988; 33(9):757-60.

[63] MarcouxS, Maheu XR, Berube S. Laparoscopic surgery in infertile with minimal or mild endometriosis. Canadian Collaboration group on endometriosis. N Engl J Med 1997; 24: 337.

[64] Bukulmez O, Yarali H, Gurgan T. The presence and extent of endometriosis do not affect clinical pregnancy and implantation rates in patients undergoing intracytoplasmic sperm injection. Eur J Obstet Gynaecol Reprod Biol. 2001; 96(1): 102-7.

[65] Hughes E, Brown J, Collins JJ, Farquhar C, Fedorkow DM, Vandekerckhove P. Ovulation suppression for endometriosis. Cochrane Database Sys Rev 2007; 18: CD 000155.

2 CONCEPT OF AETIOPATHOGENESIS OF ENDOMETRIOSIS

Kannan Kutty and Muhamed T Osman

While the precise cause of endometriosis still remains unknown and is the subject of debate, many theories have been promulgated to comprehend better and elucidate its pathogenesis .These concepts admittedly do not necessarily exclude each other. Furthermore no one theory can explicate all cases of endometriosis [1], however the concept of the aetiopathognesis seems flawed with the rapid surge of emerging molecular and proteomic profiles of diseases. It is more than gratifying to witness a revolution modifying influence on our current appreciation of the pathophysiology and etiology of endometriosis.

Theories of Pathogenesis

The pathogenesis of endometriosis has been debated and most theories fall into two broad divisions (1) Development in situ by metaplasia or (2) development as a consequence of the dissemination of endometrium [2]. The first widely considered theory of histogenesis was coelomic metaplasia; ovarian and Müllerian ducts are derived from coelomic mesothelium and it is proposed that the germinal epithelium of the ovary is responsible for endometriosis in this site [3]. This accounts for ovarian endometriosis. Endometriosis in the pelvis and peritoneum are considered to have developed from in situ metaplasia of the serosal mesothelium. However flaws in this theory exist, endometriosis has developed in women without endometrium (congenital absence of the uterus), also if coelomic metaplasia occurs in the peritoneum endometriosis would be found in men. Finally endometriosis should only then occur in sites with coelomic membranes – endometriosis has been found in every site in the body with exception of the spleen.

Sampson (1922 & 1927) [4-5] initiated the theory of retrograde menstruation in 1927, in which he proposed that menstrual effluent contained viable endometrial cells that could be transplanted to ectopic sites. Retrograde menstruation is an event seen commonly in women [6], questioned why a physiological event should frequently give rise to pathology – and yet there has been no satisfactory explanation. Other researchers [7] proved that menstrual effluent did contain viable endometrial cells by culturing tissue fragments of endometrium. In support of this theory viable endometrial cells have been found in menstrual effluent and in the peritoneal fluid, endometrium can be implanted experimentally and grown within the peritoneal cavity and thirdly the fact that all women have some degree of retrograde menstruation. Dissemination of endometrial cells through lymphatic or vascular channels may account for the finding of endometriosis at sites distant from the pelvis.

Cases of endometriosis have been documented in episiotomy and laparotomy scars following gynaecological procedures and caesarean section. Such observations suggest that ectopic endometrium can be induced iatrogenically by mechanical transplantation [8].

Since Dr. Sampson first coined the term "endometriosis" in 1921 [4-5], extensive research on pathogenesis has been carried out. Despite progress, however, no single theory has proven sufficient to explain pathogenesis satisfactorily; current concepts hold that multifactorial immune, hormonal, genetic, environmental, and anatomic factors may be responsible.

According to Sampson's theory of retrograde menstruation, during a woman's menstrual flow, some of the endometrial efflux exits the uterus via the fallopian tubes and adheres to the peritoneal surface which it invades to produce endometriosis. While most women may have some retrograde menstrual flow, normally their immune system clears the debris thwarting implantation and occurrence of endometriosis, Nevertheless, in some patients, misplaced endometrial tissue by retrograde menstruation may entrench to establish as endometriosis. Some of the possible causes that may predispose to the genesis of endometriosis include hereditary factors, toxins, or a compromised immune system. The failure of Sampson's theory to elucidate all instances of endometriosis implies that other factors such as genetic or immune differences have to be considered to explicate as to why many women with retrograde menstruation do not have endometriosis. In this context it is pertinent to quote one study that casts doubt on Sampson's theory based on finding of significant biochemical differences between endometriotic lesions and transplanted ectopic tissue [9].

Retrograde menstruation is a fairly common physiologic event .But retrograde menstruation fails to adequately elucidate the extrauterine implantation of endometrial tissue. Diagnostic laparoscopy in the perimenstrual period shows that as many as 90% of women with patent fallopian tubes have bloody peritoneal fluid. However, the increase in risk of endometriosis is associated with conditions that augment the rate of retrograde menstruation, such as congenital outflow tract obstructions. This theory is supported by various animal experiments and clinical observations support this theory [9-12].

In an attempt to verify the Samson hypothesis Thomas et al 1995 [13], conducted experiment using baboons to determine the outcome of intrapelvic injection of menstrual versus luteal endometrium on the incidence, peritoneal involvement, and stage of endometriosis, concluded that Intrapelvic injection of menstrual endometrium can induce peritoneal endometriosis and provides experimental proof favouring the Sampson hypothesis.

It was postulated that when faulty endometrium with low levels of aberrant aromatase expression reaches the pelvic peritoneum by retrograde menstruation, it excites an inflammatory response that rapidly enhances local aromatase activity (i.e., estrogen formation) induced directly or indirectly by PGs and cytokines. The retrograde flow of menstrual blood via the fallopian tubes favours internal infection or inflammation of coelomic epithelial lining leading to conversion of some peritoneal cells into endometrial cells These ectopic foci respond to cyclic hormonal fluctuations in a manner akin to intrauterine endometrium, with proliferation, secretory activity, and cyclical sloughing of menstrual products.The products of this activity, coupled with the concerted and cyclic release of cytokines and prostaglandins, induces an altered inflammatory response characterized by neovascularization and fibrosis formation. Some investigators have been able to demonstrate abnormal T- and B-cell function, abnormal complement deposition, and altered interleukin (IL)-6 production in women with endometriosis

According to Seli E and Berkkanoglu Arici AM [1] the retrograde menstruation theory is commonly accepted. Retrograde menstruation occurs in 76% to 90% of women. The much reduced occurrence of endometriosis implies that there are additional factors that predispose to endometriosis. Endometriosis is linked with alterations in both cell-mediated and humoral immunity. Impaired natural killer cell activity leading to inadequate elimination of refluxed menstrual debris may play a role in the development of endometriotic implants. Furthermore, even though the peritoneal fluid of women with endometriosis contains augmented numbers of immune cells, these appear to assist rather than hinder the formation of endometriosis. Macrophages whose function is to clear endometrial cells from the peritoneal cavity seem to enhance their proliferation by secreting growth factors and cytokines. Although it is uncertain whether these immunologic changes provoke endometriosis or are a result of its presence, they appear to play an important role in allowing endometriosis implants to persist and progress and contribute to the development of associated infertility and pelvic pain. Danazol and gonadotropin-releasing hormone (GnRH) agonists have immunomodulatory effects are commonly used for the medical therapy of endometriosis. These drugs appear to down-regulate cellular and humoral immune responses connected with their effect on endometriotic implants [1].

Coelomic Metaplasia: Meyer's theory of coelomic metaplasia is entrenched in the concept that during embryogenesis, the coelomic epithelium with multipotent cells, lining the whole pelvic cavity can become transformed into endometriotic tissue; with maturation, these cells differentiate into specific organs or tissue. Nevertheless it is implicit that these differentiated cells can become "dedifferentiated", and result in a new kind of tissue or organ This phenomenon is illustrated by the dedifferentiation of the cells that envelop the ovaries, to become endometrial cells.. Thus, these transformed endometrial cells on the ovary are subject to cyclic changes with menstruation, corresponding to its normal complement in the uterus. While the implantation and the metaplasia theories illustrate the mechanism of the initiation of endometriotic lesions, they do not explain the diverse clinical profile of endometriosis.

The metaplasia theory implies that under different influences, coelomic tissue could be transformed into endometrium. However, there has been no documented direct proof of the genesis of endometrial stroma at the conclusion of the metaplastic process. Furthermore this theory signifies that ectopic endometrium arises in situ from local tissues, including germinal epithelium of the ovary and remnants of the Müllerian and Wolffian ducts. Furthermore this theory implies that the origin of peritoneal endometriosis is from in situ metaplasia of totipotent mesothelial serosal cells. The predominance of endometriosis in females and hardly occurs in males, casts shadow of doubt on the conception of metaplasia to explain endometriosis.

Inflammation possibly triggers the change of one type of cell to the other [14]. At this juncture it is pertinent to delve further on the role of inflammation. Numerous cytokines including interleukin (IL)-1, 6, 8, 10, tumor necrosis factor (TNF)-alpha, and vascular endothelial growth factor (VEGF) were reported to be increased in the peritoneal fluid (PF) of women with endometriosis. Those cytokines may be concerned with macrophage activation, involved in inflammatory change and enhanced angiogenesis. Nevertheless reduced expression of some cytokines such as IL-2, and interferon (IFN)-gamma.was also found... They signify disturbed T- and natural killer (NK)-cell function. Endometriotic implants generate some factors, such as matrix metalloproteinases (MMPs), and Bcl-2, and impact their capacity to lodge in the peritoneum.Peritoneal cytokines, originating from mesothelial cells, leukocytes and ectopic endometrial cells, interact locally and systemically in women with endometriosis.

Yet another facet worth considering is the vital role of p38 mitogen-activated protein kinase (MAPK) in the process of inflammation is well recognized. Inflammation is conceived as an etiological factor for endometriosis Osamu Yoshino, et al 2006 [15], assessed in BALB/c mice, the outcome of FR 167653,(a p38 MAPK inhibitor), on the genesis of endometriosis. The estradiol-treated ovariectomized Balb/c mice representing endometriosis model, were injected intraperitoneally with small pieces of endometrial tissues of the syngenic donor mice. The animals were injected with either 30 mg/kg FR 167653 or only vehicle (control) s.c. twice a day, starting 2 days previous to endometrial injection. At the end of three weeks, the examination of peritoneal fluids and the induced endometriotic lesions.showed that the weight of all the endometriotic lesions per mouse and the levels of interleukin-6 and monocyte chemoattractant protein-1 in the peritoneal fluid were notably lesser in the FR 167653-treated mice relative to that in the control mice. These observations imply the inhibitory effect of FR 167653 on the development of endometriosis probably by suppressed peritoneal inflammation [15].

Both Sampson retrograde menstruation, and implantation and the metaplasia theory focus upon the implantation/metaplasia of cells, and thus on subtle lesions, i.e. small initial lesions, which will subsequently grow and develop to more severe disease. These theories are attractive because of the abundance of data demonstrating retrograde menstruation as a frequent phenomenon occurring almost in all women, the presence in peritoneal fluid of viable endometrial cells, which have the capacity to implant, to grow and to infiltrate superficially. According to this view, the development into a more severe condition may be influenced by a decreased cellular immunity, a lower NK cell activity, peritoneal fluid cytokines and growth factors, or low peritoneal fluid steroid concentrations in the luteal phase [16].

These theories are attractive since each step in the pathophysiology has been documented. It is important to recognize that this theory, cannot explain why progression occurs in some women only. Fundamentally this theory holds that progression of endometriosis once established is unavoidable, albeit at a different speed and to a different stage according to modulating factors. Essentially, this theory considers endometriosis as normal endometrial cells which behave abnormally, because of the abnormal environment, i.e. the peritoneal milieu. This is however, not supported by all [16-17]. The key event in the process is implantation or metaplasia, which thus has been the subject of many investigations, and the early subtle lesions become very important.

The endometriotic disease theory considers retrograde menstruation, viable endometrial cells in peritoneal fluid, and occasional implantation of some of these cells a normal physiological phenomenon. These non-implanted and implanted cells are normally removed by the defense mechanisms of the body such as macrophages [18].

Attachment and implantation is favourized when the mesothelial layer is damaged by trauma, infection or even by low grade inflammation, e.g. irritation caused by CO_2 pneumoperitoneum, or by abundant retrograde menstruation. It also seems logical that attachment and implantation must occur more frequently when more viable cells are present in peritoneal fluid. Although these cells can temporarily grow and develop depending upon the environment, their ultimate fate when left alone will be their spontaneous disappearance. This can result in some fibrotic or scar tissue as the remnant of local inflammation, containing eventually some endometrial cells, shielded from the blood stream and immunocompetent cells comparable to the bacteria in an abscess [16,18].

The much lower prevalence of endometriosis implies that other factors determine propensity to endometriosis Notwithstanding this theory has its pros and cons An observation that endorses this theory is the increased incidence of endometriosis in women with augmented retrograde menstruation as they menstruate more frequently or have a congenitally absent cervix. Retrograde menstruation via the fallopian tubes into the peritoneal cavity is a very frequent physiologic occurrence in all menstruating women with patent tubes. Although approximately 90% of women may have some degree of retrograde menstruation not all develop endometriosis [19]. This has engendered another hypothesis that women with endometriosis have reduced immunological clearance of misplaced endometrial cells within the peritoneal cavity.

Some of the possible causes that may predispose to

the genesis of endometriosis include hereditary factors, toxins, or a compromised immune system. The downside of this theory is its failure to elucidate all instances of endometriosis; hence this implies that other factors such as genetic or immune differences have to be hypothesized to explain as to why many women with retrograde menstruation do not have endometriosis. In this context it is pertinent to quote one study that casts doubt on Sampson's theory based on finding of significant biochemical differences between endometriotic lesions and transplanted ectopic tissue.

Role of Estrogens:

Endometriosis being an estrogen-dependent condition is seen primarily during the reproductive years. In experimental models, estrogen is necessary to induce or maintain endometriosis. Medical therapy is often targeted at lowering estrogen levels to contain the disease. Additionally, research on aromatase, an estrogen-synthesizing enzyme, has provided evidence for the continuation of endometriosis after menopause and hysterectomy.

Endometriosis, as already stated earlier develops mostly in women of reproductive age and regresses after menopause or ovariectomy, signifying that the growth is estrogen-dependent [20].

In experimental models, estrogen is necessary to induce or maintain endometriosis. Obviously medical therapy is often intended to reduce estrogen levels to manage the disease. Additionally, the current research focus on aromatase, an estrogen-synthesizing enzyme, has amply proved the pathogenesis of endometriosis after menopause and hysterectomy. Aromatase P450 (P450arom), the key enzyme for biosynthesis of estrogen, is a vital hormone for the genesis and development of endometriosis. No obvious aromatase activity is present in normal endometrium, hence estrogen is not locally formed in endometrium. On the contrary endometriotic tissue, is rich with extremely elevated levels of aromatase [21], which stimulates substantial production of estrogen. In addition prostaglandin, an important mediator of inflammation appreciably induces aromatase activity producing in turn local estrogen in this tissue. Estrogen also stimulates cyclo-oxygenase-2 augmenting the formation of prostaglandin E_2 in endometriosis [21].

Serdar E. Bulun et al 2004 [21], have demonstrated an "intracrine" effect of estrogen in uterine leiomyomas and endometriosis: Estrogen produced by aromatase activity in the cytoplasm of leiomyoma smooth muscle cells or endometriotic stromal cells can affect by readily binding to its nuclear receptor within the same cell [22-24].

In contrast, normal endometrium and myometrium, are deficient in aromatase expression [23-24]. Aromatase catalyzes the conversion of androstenedione and testosterone to estrone and estradiol. The gene that encodes this enzyme is articulated in numerous human tissue cells including ovarian granulosa cells, adipose tissue, skin, fibroblasts, and the brain. As is well known in woman of reproductive-age the ovary is the principal organ for estrogen biosynthesis, and this takes place in a cyclic fashion. Upon binding of follicle-stimulating hormone (FSH) to its G-protein-coupled receptor in the granulosa cell membrane, intracellular cyclic adenosine monophosphate (cAMP) levels increase and enhance binding of two critical transcription factors [i.e., steroidogenic factor-1 (SF-1) and cAMP response element binding protein (CREB)], to the typically sited proximal promoter II of the aromatase gene [25-26]. This, in turn, activates aromatase expression and consequently estrogen secretion from the preovulatory follicle [26].

Alternatively, in postmenopausal women, estrogen formation occurs in the adipose tissue and skin [27-29]. Contrary to cAMP regulation of aromatase expression in the ovary, this is controlled mainly by cytokines [interleukin (IL)-6, IL-11, tumor necrosis factor alpha (TNFα)] and glucocorticoids via the alternative use of promoter I.4 in adipose tissue and skin fibroblasts [30]. The key substrate for aromatase in adipose tissue and skin is androstenedione from adrenals. In postmenopausal women, ~2% of circulating androstenedione is converted to estrone, which is further changed to estradiol in these peripheral tissues.

Extensive and intensive studies on aromatase expression in endometriosis [31-32], revealed exceedingly elevated levels of aromatase mRNA in extraovarian endometriotic implants and endometriomas. In addition endometriosis-derived stromal cells in culture incubated with a cAMP analog exhibited exceptionally high levels of aromatase activity [33] Further investigations on stimulators of aromatase activity via a cAMP-dependent pathway in endometriosis revealed that Prostaglandin E_2 (PGE_2) as the most powerful inducer of aromatase activity in endometriotic stromal cells [33]. Mediated via the cAMP-inducing EP_2 receptor subtype additionally, estrogen was found to enhance PGE_2 formation by stimulating cyclooxygenase type 2 (COX-2) enzyme in endometrial stromal cells in culture [34]. The establishment of constant local production of estrogen and prostaglandins (PGs), leads to the proliferative and inflammatory features of endometriosis Aromatase micro RNA was detected in the eutopic endometrial samples of women with moderate to severe endometriosis and absent in disease-free women albeit in much lesser quantities relative to endometriotic implants. This weak finding in the eutopic endometrium may imply a genetic fault in women with endometriosis It is postulated by Serdar E. Bulun et al, that when faulty endometrium with low levels of aberrant aromatase expression reaches the pelvic peritoneum by retrograde menstruation, it excites an inflammatory response that rapidly enhances local aromatase activity (i.e., estrogen formation) induced directly or indirectly by PGs and cytokines [32]. The clinical relevance of aromatase expression is best appreciated if aromatase inhibitors could be of benefit in the treatment of endometriosis. In addition to aberrant aromatase expression other important factors in molecular mechanism may be involved in the pathogenesis of pelvic endometriosis ;these factors may include 1) abnormal expression of matrix metalloproteinases, tissue inhibitor of metalloproteinase-, 2) certain cytokines (IL-6, RANTES (regulated on activation, normal T cell expressed and secreted), and 3) epidermal growth factor [35-36]. Furthermore another proposal for the genesis of endometriosis has been suggested. That pinpoints to a flawed immune system that fails to eliminate peritoneal surfaces of the retrograde menstrual flow the development of endometriosis [37].

Undeniably the endometriotic lesions have estrogen receptors (ER) as well as aromatase, that catalyses the conversion of androgens to estrogens, signifying that local estrogen production may fuel the growth of lesions. It is notable that the expression patterns of ER and progesterone receptors in endometriotic lesions are different from those in the eutopic endometrium. Additionally estrogen metabolism, including the expression pattern of aromatase and the regulation of 17 beta-hydroxysteroid dehydrogenase type 2 (an enzyme responsible for the inactivation of estradiol to estrone), is changed in the eutopic endometrium of women with endometriosis, adenomyosis, and/or leiomyomas compared to that in the eutopic endometrium of normal women. Immunostaining for P450arom in endometrial biopsy specimens diagnosed these diseases with sensitivity and specificity of 91 and 100%, respectively. This is valuable in the clinical diagnosis of endometriosis. The polymorphisms in the ER-alpha gene, the CYP19 gene encoding aromatase, and several other genes are linked with the risk of endometriosis. Studies focusing on these will lead to better understanding of the etiopathogensis of endometriosis [38]. That estrogen has a vital role in the immune response in immune-mediated diseases hardly needs any reiteration. Estrogen receptors are expressed in a variety of immunocompetent cells, including CD4(+) and CD8(+) T cells and macrophages Based on a distinct profile of cytokine production, data accrued hitherto have shown modulatory effects for estrogen on the TH1-type and TH2-type cells, which signify two distinctly clear cut forms of the effector specific immune response. Recent evidence indicates that estrogens inhibit the production of TH1 proinflammatory cytokines, such as IL-12, TNF-alpha and IFN-gamma; on the contrary estrogens encourage the generation of TH2 anti-inflammatory cytokines, such as IL-10, IL-4, and TGF-beta.

Salem ML, 2004 [39], postulated that estrogen aggravates or suppresses inflammatory diseases mediated by skewing TH1-type to TH2-type response. This view conceptualizes a novel mechanism for the modulatory impact of estrogen on certain inflammatory diseases that can result in useful or unfavorable outcomes depending on the type of immune response involved.

Role of other hormones

While we have drawn our attention to estrogens and their role in endometriosis it is essential to focus on the role of other hormones in the pathogenesis of this disorder. It is known that the periodic expression of matrix metalloproteinases (MMPs) by human endometrium has been implicated to play a part in the invasive process essential to set up endometriosis. Progesterone can inhibit endometrial MMP-3 and MMP-7 expression and this requires the local action of TGFβ and may also be associated with the local generation of retinoic acid by stromal cells. A constant expression of several MMPs in endometriotic lesions has been reported, indicating a failure of progesterone or locally produced factors to suppress these enzymes. This leads us to focus on the therapeutic relevance of Progestins which are effective in endometriosis but, the precise mechanisms of their action still remain unresolved. The investigative studies of Verena Mönckedieck,et al 2009 [40], are worthy of mention. They throw light on the role of progesterone in endometriosis. They studied employing nude mice, the impact of different progestins on notable features of extracellular matrix degradation and angiogenesis implicated in the setting up and continuation of ectopic endometrial lesions. The study involved intraperitoneal transplantation of human endometrium into nude mice. Following one week and four weeks of treatment with progesterone, dydrogesterone, or its metabolite dihydrodydrogesterone, respectively, they evaluated ectopic lesions for proliferation and apoptosis expression of estrogen receptor α, progesterone receptor-AB, the angiogenetic factors, cysteine-rich angiogenic inducer (CYR61), basic fibroblast growth factor (bFGF), vascular endothelial growth factor (VEGFA) and the matrix metalloproteinase (MMP)-2, -3, -7 and -9. In addition functional influence on angiogenesis was also assessed .Even though dydrogesterone appreciably reduced proliferation of endometrial stromal cells the end of four weeks, suppression of apoptosis was unrelated to progestins. While all progestins substantially reduced expression of MMP-2 and dydrogesterone reduced MMP-3. In the grafted endometrial tissue, progesterone and dihydrodydrogesterone, suppressed transcription of bFGF and VEGFA and CYR61 were suppressed by dihydrodydrogesterone and dydrogesterone. Microvessel density was slightly suppressed by progestins, while number of stabilized vessels increased. Thus, progestins control factors vital for the genesis and continuance of ectopic endometrial lesions [40].

It is of interest at this juncture to allude to the role of MMP and TIMP in mediating the survival and implantation of endometrial cells in the peritoneal fluid. Matrix metalloproteinases (MMPs) have play a part in the degradation and turnover of extracellular matrix proteins and their action is regulated by specific tissue inhibitors called tissue inhibitors of metalloproteinases (TIMPs). In a study comparing the concentrations of total and active MMP-9 in peritoneal fluid of 22 infertile men with mild or moderate endometriosis and those with those in a control group of 21.infertile patients it was found that the mean total concentrations of MMP-9 in the peritoneal fluid of patients with endometriosis was almost thrice higher (6.2 ± 1.8 ng/ml), compared to the concentration of 2.9 ± 2.6 ng/ml in the control group .There was no significant difference in the levels of active MMP-9 between the groups. The concentrations of TIMP-1, were appreciably lower in endometriotic peritoneal fluids than in peritoneal fluid of control women,(1.02 ± 0.21 ng/ml and 1.16 ± 0.18 ng/ml respectively. Neither was any correlation between stage of disease, steroid hormone concentration, MMP-9 (total and active) and TIMP-1 was found. Thus their findings imply that the disequilibrium between MMP-9 and TIMP-1 in peritoneal fluid of women with endometriosis may play a significant role in the pathogenesis of the disease [41]. On reaching the peritoneal cavity, the survival and implantation of endometrial cells seem to be mediated by abnormal MMP and TIMP expression, altered immune milieu, aberrant local aromatase activity, and genetic and environmental factors [42].

Müllerianosis: Another theory proposes that cells with the potential to differentiate into endometrial cells are laid down in paths that during embryonic development and organogenesis. These tracts follow the Mullerian tract as it moves caudally at 8–10 weeks of embryonic life. Primitive endometrial cells become displaced from the migrating uterus and act like stem cells. This theory is supported by foetal autopsy. Müllerianosis is exactly the condition of "developmentally misplaced endometrial tissue," [43].

Batt RE, et al 2007 [43], defined it as an organoid structure of embryonic descent a choristoma made up of müllerian rests--normal endometrium, normal endosalpinx, and normal endocervix--singly or in combination, included within other normal organs during organogenesis.. Histologically, endometrial-müllerianosis and endometriosis both comprise endometrial glands and stroma, Notwithstanding both these conditions have different pathogenesis. Batt RE, et al 1990 [44] suggested that müllerianosis is a distinctive form of endometriosis, which differs in its pathogenesis from all forms of transplantation endometriosis be it of lymphatic, hematogenous, transtubal, or iatrogenic origin; it is also separate from endometriosis of coelomic metaplasia [44].

Müllerianosis' has borad connotation to in clue collection of epithelial and mesenchymal 'metaplasias' and proliferations that are usual in the female peritoneal cavity, commonly around the pelvic viscera and particularly the ovaries. In many ways, their morphological features identical to their cellular analogues lining or forming the müllerian duct derivatives, such as endosalpinx (the fallopian tube mucosal lining), endometrium,and smooth muscle It is pertinent to refer to Sampson's classification of misplaced endometrial or müllerian tissue into "four or possibly five groups, on the basis of the manner this tissue deposited at ectopic site. Sampson [5] classified aberrant or misplaced endometrial tissue on the grounds of its pathogenesis: 1) direct or primary endometriosis [adenomyosis]; an analogous form occurs in the wall of the fallopian tube from its mucosal incursion [endosalpingiosis]; 2) peritoneal or implantation endometriosis; 3) transplantation endometriosis; 4) metastatic endometriosis; and 5) developmentally misplaced endometrial tissue [4-5].

In vitro study of secretion profile of IL and growth factors (VEGF, IGF-I, TGFbeta) by endometrial tissues and endometrioid heterotopies in patients with external genital endometriosis revealed enhanced production of IL-1beta, IL-2, IL-6, and VEGF in the endometrium in severe external genital endometriosis, and decreased secretion of TGFbeta; but just the opposite profile was seen in endometrioid foci. In all probability local cytokine imbalance and enhanced proliferative activity of endometrial cells are implicated in the pathogenesis of endometrioid foci. Other than the role of interleukins and growth factors referred to above in the genesis of endometriosis the importance of c-myc protooncogene and its polypeptide product significant regulator of cell proliferation and differentiation in the pathogenesis of endometriosis.was explored.It is assumed ovarian steroids promote growth of different uterine cell types through altered expression of the c-myc gene. With the aim to verify this assumption whether c-myc expression may also be involved in the genesis and growth of endometriosis, Schenken RS, et al 1991 [45], evaluated c-myc expression in eutopic and ectopic endometrial tissue from women undergoing surgery for endometriosis. Immunocytochemical studies revealed positive staining for c-myc protein in both glandular cytoplasm and nuclei and only stromal cell nuclei, in both eutopic and ectopic endometrium. This finding impies that c-myc expression may be a key controller of cell proliferation in endometriotic tissue.

Angiogenesis

While various theories attempt to elucidate the occurrence of extrauterine endometrial tissue, none of them can either satisfactorily explain all disease locations and appearances or the manner these fragments establish into endometriotic lesions [46]. It is relevant at this juncture to allude the release of VEGF along with IL 6810 and TNF which are all increased in peritoneal fluid of women with endometriosis [14].

Obviously angiogenesis is possibly with VEGF. New vessel formation has long been recognized as a feature of endometriosis, often clearly visible at laparoscopy. Recent work has focused on identifying the role of vascularization in the pathogenesis of endometriosis, by allowing lesions to establish and grow [46].

This theory is further fortified by laboratory documentation of this conversion. In vitro experimental model of endometriosis employing human ovarian surface epithelial cells supports the metaplastic origin of endometriotic lesions from the ovarian surface epithelium. The model of Matsuura K, et al [47], entailimg coculture of both ovarian surface epithelium and ovarian stromal cells with 17beta estradiol revealed that the ovarian surface epithelium cells produced a luminal structure, encircled by endometrial stromal cells with an epithelial mesenchymal structure.That endometriosis may result from a sequential transformation from the adjacent mesothelial cells is further confirmed by immunopositivity of epithelial membrane antigen and cytokeratin in the glandular cells and cilia, as well as in the microvilli coupled with the EM findings of tight junctions on cell surfaces [47].

The autoimmune theory of endometriosis

Before we go to specific issue of the autoimmune etiology of endometriosis it will useful to recapitulate briefly the concept of autoimmune diseases. Majority of autoimmune diseases occur in women, and these are most commonly in reproductive age group. The reasons for this higher gender predominance are still unclear, some autoimmune diseases occur more often in postmenopausal women. It is of interest to note that while in some cases pregnancy has an ameliorating influence on this disease while in others it is aggravated by pregnancy.There may exacerbations of the illness following delivery.

As for its etiology it is possibly multifactorial involving genetics, environmental and hormonal factors. The disease has a genetic basis as it is seen as clusters in certain families. Different members of a family can have varying types of autoimmune diseases.

The pathogenesis of autoimmune diseases and autoimmune reactions

Autoimmune reactions can be triggered in several ways:

- A substance in the body that is normally strictly contained in a specific area (and thus is hidden from the immune system) is released into the general circulation. For example, the fluid in the eyeball is normally contained within the eyeball's chambers. If a blow to the eye releases this fluid into the bloodstream, the immune system may react against it.

- A normal body substance is altered. For example, viruses, drugs, sunlight, or radiation may change a protein's structure in a way that makes it seem foreign.

- The immune system responds to a foreign substance that is similar in appearance to a natural body substance and inadvertently targets the body substance as well as the foreign substance.

Something malfunctions in the cells that control antibody production. For example, cancerous B lymphocytes may produce abnormal antibodies that attack red blood cells

Having briefly dealt with the fringe of the problem of broad aspect of autoimmune diseases we shall consider some of the current concepts with regards to autoimmune nature of endometriosis.

The intriguing question is endometriosis an autoimmune aiseases question apart we shall consider some of the known aspects of the disease. The link between antiendometrial anibodies and endometriosis will be touched upon here. An important factor in the pathogenesis and progression of endometriosis could be attributed to, a failure in the immune system tolerance to self-antigens, resulting in an autoimmune condition. The detection of antiendometrial antibodies both in peritoneal fluid and serum of women with endometriosis is an undeniable proof for this autoimmune phenomenon. The spectrum of autoimmune alterations comprises a decrease in NK activity, increased generation of proinflammatory cytokines, and enhanced angiogenic activity. Additionally the striking similarity between the immunological profiles in experimentally induced endometriosis in a Wistar rat model and those seen in human, is noteworthy [48].

Apart from antiendometrial antibodies other antibodies such as antinuclear antibody.and lupus anticoagfulant antibody have been found in endometriosis patients Besides immunoglobulin IgG autroantibodies,and IgM autoantibodies have also been found in patients with endometriosis. Among IgG autoantibodies, those to phospholipids were most common, followed in order of frequency by antibodies to histones and nucleotides. The incidence of IgM autoantibodies was reversed, with antinucleotides appearing most frequently and antiphospholipids least frequently. These findings imply that endometriosis is linked with abnormal polyclonal B cell activation, a typical feature of autoimmune disease. This argument is further fortified by the elevated levels immunoglobulin (principally IgG) in patients with endometriosis, and more so in lupus anticoagulant-positive than lupus anticoagulant-negative endometriosis patients.

Among 59 laparoscopically staged endometriosis patients, 28.8% tested positive for antinuclear antibody. Of 44 patients, 45.5% were lupus anticoagulant positive (greater than 1.3) and 20.5% were within a borderline range (1.2-1.3). Antinuclear antibody positivity was inversely related to stage of disease ($P = .009$); lupus anticoagulant positivity exhibited a similar trend, but did not reach statistical significance. Of 31 endometriosis patients, 64.5% exhibited immunoglobulin G (IgG) autoantibodies and 45.2% demonstrated IgM autoantibodies to at least one of 16 antigens investigated. Among IgG autoantibodies, those to phospholipids were most frequently detected, followed in order of frequency by antibodies to histones and nucleotides. The incidence of IgM autoantibodies was inverted, with antinucleotides appearing most frequently and antiphospholipids least frequently. A strong correlation was noted between the presence of lupus anticoagulant and antinuclear antibody with both IgG and IgM autoantibodies. These observations suggest that endometriosis is associated with abnormal polyclonal B cell activation, a typical feature of autoimmune disease. The elevated immunoglobulin levels (particularly IgG) in patients with endometriosis, further support this contention and more so in lupus anticoagulant-positive than lupus anticoagulant-negative endometriosis patients

The following may further illustrate the relevance of the theory of autoimmune nature of endometriosis. In addition it is to be appreciated that a mosaic of antibodies has added to the myriad complexities of the undeniably complicated disease.Just to illustrate briefly the type of antibodies we have cited some of the following.

In investigating immunoglobulins IgG, IgA and IgM against endometrial antigens in patients with endometriosis and fertile controls were tested IgG, IgA, or IgM in endometrium, serum, and peritoneal fluid (PF) of the patients and controls using Western blot analysis. Mathur S,et al 1990 [49], observed the presence of endogenous IgG in 78% of the endometria or endometriosis implants from the patients and 22% of the endometria from the controls and endometrial IgA and IgM were detectable in few controls and patients. Further it was observed that IgG in the serum and/or PF of patients with endometriosis was specifically aimed at only certain antigens (i.e.with molecular weights of 34, 42, 82, 94, 110, 120, and 140 kd) found in the patients' endometrium or endometriosis implants. IgA and IgM in the serum or PF of the patients and controls were nonspecific in their reactivity. Endometrial antigens in endometrium or endometriotic implants of patients with endometriosis, and drawing IgG responses, may be applicable to and consistent with autoimmunity in endometriosis [49].

The identification of endometrial antigens provoking autoimmunity would establish an antibody assay which would serve both as a non-invasive diagnostic test as well as a monitoring aid in clinical assessment of endometriosis. With this objective Pillai S etal, [50], performed systematic study of Forty-six women with endometriosis, 4 women with uterine leiomyomata, 4 with pelvic adhesions, 3 with repeat Cesarean sections (conditions that coexist with or predispose to endometriosis) and 46 controls. The investigations comprising Two-dimensional gel electrophoresis of endometrial extracts, Western blot analysis, passive hemagglutination and enzyme-linked immunosorbent assay (ELISA), amino acid sequencing and molecular studies on chosen antigens revealed that endometriosis patients had appreciable IgG antibodies to two endometrial antigens transferrin and alpha 2-HS-glycoprotein. The highlight of this study is the diagnostic value of an antibody assay using these antigens for diagnosing endometriosis [50].

Prompted by the objective to explore the presence and clinical correlation of serum autoantibodies to carbonic anhydrase (CA) in women with and without endometriosis. D'Cruz OJ,et al 1996 [51], tested sera of 319 patients with laproscopically diagnosed pelvic endomertiosis in varying stages ,100 with other gynecologic problems and 100 control women. Positive sera also were systematically tested for antiendometrial antibodies and antinuclear antibodies (ANA) antibodies to single-stranded (ss) and double-stranded (ds) DNA, and extractable nuclear antigens (Sm, nRNP, Ro, and La). The study revealed that; a)a subgroup of patients with endometriosis had autoantibodies to native and linear epitopes of the CA protein, b) occurrence of anti-CA antibodies was linked with antiendometrial antibodies and ANA.and c) Anti-CA antibodies were allied with a higher prognostic value of the disease when all patient subgroups were considered together [51].

Another investigative study of the connection of rheumatoid arthritis-associated single nucleotide polymorphisms in endometriosis.merits mentioned. It revealed an association of CCL21 (rs2812378) and HLA-DRB1 (rs660895) with moderate to severe endometriosis [52].

It is suggested that the pathogenesis of endometriosis involves abnormal immunologic mechanism Fc receptor-like 3 gene (FCRL3) has been projected as a novel autoimmune predisposing factor. Prompted by hypothesis of a probable association between endometriosis, infertility and FCRL3 polymorphisms. The authors conducted a case-control study comprising 170 women with endometriosis-related infertility, 91 women with idiopathic infertility and 166 controls. Using TaqMan PCR, they performed detection of FCRL3 polymorphisms (-169C/T, -110G/A, +358C/G and +1381A/G). Systematic statistrical analysis of the single-marker analysis revealed that FCRL3-169C/T was appreciably coupled with endometriosis (p=0.004), irrespective of the stage of the disease, p=0.011 and p=0.035, respectively [52].

Another theory has it that the normal occurrence of endometrial reflux in the fallopian tubes during menstruation may, in some circumstances, surmount local defense mechanisms, implant, and proliferate. Nevertheless, the presence of endometriosis in sites far removed from pelvic organs led to the quest for other theories such as genetic background, embryonic rest theory and stem cell dysfunction: The stem cell theory does not only substantiate the findings of endometriosis at distant sites away from the peritoneal cavity,but also elucidates resistance to some treatments, and the infrequently occurs even after hysterectomy. Recently, it was demonstrated that bone marrow–derived (mesenchymal) stem cells could lead to expression of endometriosis in a mouse model [53].

Another study demonstrated how endometriosis was initiated from stem cells, in a mouse model whose uterus was removed so that endometriosis could not originate from endometrial cells (either through retrograde menstruation, or hematogenous or lymphatic dissemination). In their experimental model, stem cells populated endometriotic implants, leading to disease progression. They observed the presence of stem cells in nearly every one of the organs of the body including the peritoneal cavity and uterus.

With a view to confirm the proposition of the existence of a likely endometriosis inducing factor(s) (EIF) in the blood of women with endometriosis. Rasheed K,et al [53], investigated fifteen women of each three different degrees of endometriosis and fifteen women without endometriosis as a control group. The women sera were co-cultured with mesenchymal stem cells (MSCs) which were followed up weekly to look for morphological changes and to detect Annexin 1 marker and ß-actin gene by reverse transcriptase polymerase chain reaction. MSCs cultured with sera of all cases regardless of the severity of endometriosis, exhibited morphological alterations resembling endometrial like cells and glands- by the 4th week in 60%, 60% & 100% respectively. These cells were seen from the first week in women with moderate and severe types (20% for each group). There proportion of the transformation into endometrial like cells augmented in an ascending order among the three groups where it was 30±25.8%, 45±29.9% and 75±37.9% respectively. Additionally number of endometrial like cells detected weekly, are found increasing with the severity of disease is. There was no change in any of the cultures of serum of the control group Besides, with progressive differentiation the density of stem cells decreased substantially.and the differentiated cells expressed the Annexin-1 marker.: These data evidently support that serum of women with endometriosis has a factor(s) that induces the alteration of the MSCs into endometrial like cells and glands in vitro. This finding not only substantiate a new theory for the etiology of endometriosis but also may have a potential implication on the therapy of this debilitating condition [53].

Endometriosis is tacitly supposed to be a progressive disease, with inevitable growth and development of lesions once the disease has set in According to a novel concept the transition of endometriosis to endometriotic disease is regarded as identical to the origin and evolution of a benign tumour. This conception obviously implicates cellular alterations such as mutations. According to this theory endometriosis develops from endometriotic cells that have 'escaped' the influence of protective and regulatory factors in the peritoneal fluid [18].

In this context it is pertinent to allude to the the possible role of the immune system which can recognize and eliminate altered or misplaced autologous cells such as ectopic endometrial cells. This mechanism may operate in most women, preventing the development of endometriosis. Functional alterations of cells of the immune system in women with endometriosis have been observed; these functional changes affect monocytes/macrophages, natural killer cells, cytotoxic T-lymphocytes and B cells. In the light of these observations in women with endometriosis it is probable that these changes involve diminished surveillance, recognition and obliteration of the ectopic endometrial cells and potential facilitation of their implantation and development of endometriosis. Peripheral blood monocytes (PBM) and peritoneal macrophages (PM) may play a key role in this regard, and may control function of other immune cells. Dmowski WP et al 1996 [54], have shown that in normal fertile women without endometriosis, PBM and PM repress endometrial cell proliferation in vitro. In endometriosis, PBM stimulate and PM inhibit endometrial cell proliferation and the cytotoxic effect of PM is inversely correlated with the stage of the disease. The decrease in PM cytotoxic function is controlled by prostaglandin synthesis. In infertile women without endometriosis, the effects of PM and PBM are variable. In about a third of patients, the effects of PM and PBM suggest subclinical endometriosis; in the remaining patients the effects of PM and PBM are similar to those of fertile controls. It is noteworthy that endometrial cells in women with endometriosis are more sensitive to the stimulatory effect of PBM, and more resistant to the cytotoxicity of the immune cells [54].

At this juncture it seems relevant to make reference also to the association of p53 polymorphisms with endometriosis impelled by the aim of assessing the link between endometriosis and the p53 polymorphism. Chi Chen Chang,.et al 2002 [55], conducted a prospective study enrolling 118 women with and 140 without endometriosis. The former were grouped as those with moderate or severe endometriosis and the other without endometriosis. By Polymerase chain reaction p53 codon 72 polymorphisms (arginine homozygosity, heterozygosity, and proline homozygosity) was detected. The evaluation of relations between endometriosis and p53 polymorphisms observed that the distributions of diverse p53 polymorphisms differed remarkably between groups. The endometriosis group showed level of 10.2%, 66.9%, and 22.9% respectively arginine homozygotes, heterozygotes, and proline homozygotes and 30.7%, 50%, and 19.3% in the group without endometriosis. In addition to the findings of the association of endometriosis with p53 polymorphism.it was found that p53 arginine homozygotes have reduced risk for endometriosis while Heterozygotes and proline homozygotes are exposed to increased risk for endometriosis [55].

Further, it is of interest to quote the observations of Vercellini P, et al 1994 on the analysis of p53 and ras gene mutations in endometriosis. Variceli et al 1994 [56], reported that no activating mutations in codons 12, 13 and 61 of ras genes nor inactivating mutations in exons 5-9 of the p53 tumor suppressor gene were detected by polymerase chain reaction and single-strand conformation polymorphism methods in either eutopic or ectopic endometrium from 10 women with severe endometriosis [56].

Molecular Aspects of Endometriosis:

Research also showed that exogeneous Annexin-1 can protect cells from necrosis induced by hydrogen peroxide [57]. Thus, increased Annexin-1 levels may inhibit the necrosis of refluxed endometrial cells and keep them viable, which is necessary for the development of endometriosis [58]. Annexin-1 functions as a substrate for the EGF receptor tyrosine kinase, which has a significant role in cell proliferation and differentiation [59]. Additionally, it holds phosphorylation sites for significant proliferative signaling molecules, including several signal transducing kinase associated hepatocyte growth factor receptor [60], and protein kinase C [61]. The overexpression of Annexin-1 may promote the proliferation of endometrial cells by modulating these signal transduction pathways [58].

The relation between Annexin-1 and the immune system and its expression in the peritoneal fluids possibly may render the peritoneal micromelieu conducive for implantation and growth of refluxed endometrial cells leading to endometriosis. Endometriosis, is known as a local pelvic inflammatory disorder.. It has been shown that macrophages in the peritoneal fluid participate dynamically in the start, upkeep and evolution of endometriosis [62]. Changes in T cell-mediated immunity take place in patients with endometriosis [61]. It has been shown that Annexin-1 has many functions attributed to it ;it controls activities of both the innate and adaptive immune cells such as macrophages and T lymphocytes,and regulates the phagocytic potential of macrophages and its production of TNF-α and IL-6., Annexin 1 derived peptides suppress antigen-driven cellular proliferation and cytokine production. Annexin-1 augments anti-CD3/CD28- mediated CD25 and CD69 expression, and increases the activation and proliferation of T cells in response to anti-CD3 plus anti-CD28 stimulation. Elevated levels of Annexin-1 in both endometrium and in peritoneal fluids may alter the components of the peritoneal fluids and the local immune microenvironment.Thus endometriosis may develop once a defective "disposal system" allows the implantation and growth of endometrial cells or fragments [60]. Thus, the overexpression of Annexin-1 in eutopic endometrium, and its presence in the peritoneal fluids of women with endometriosis, might increase the survival and proliferation of refluxed endometrial cells, and may also make the pelvic environment become "permissive" to their adherence and implantation.

Chun found from their study, expression of Annexin-1 protein mostly in endometrial glandular cells during the menstrual cycle,signifying that Annexin-1 may act on endometrial glandular and the stromal cells by autocrine or paracrine mechanisms, without significant change with the hormone levels. The actual mechanism of Annexin-1 on endometrial cells warrant further investigation [58].

Cytokines and endometriosis:

From an extensive review it was obvious that numerous cytokines including interleukin (IL)-1, 6, 8, 10, tumor necrosis factor (TNF)-α, and vascular endothelial growth factor (VEGF) were found enhanced in the peritoneal fluid (PF) of women with endometriosis. These cytokines are possibly concerned with in macrophage activation, inflammatory change and augmented angiogenesis. Nevertheless, some cytokines such as IL-2, and interferon (IFN)-γ.were less expressed. They signify the impaired T- and natural killer (NK)-cell function. Endometriotic implants generate some factors, e.g. matrix metalloproteinases (MMPs), Bcl-2, and upset their potential to implant into the peritoneum. There is, a local and systemic, interplay between cytokines and leucocytes and endometrial cells in women with endometriosis. Further studies about the specific role and interactions of these cytokines are warranted to enhance the understanding of endometriosis in order to develop newl therapies [14].

The TNF-alpha concentration in the peritoneal fluid considerably correlated with the menstrual cycle day (P < 0.01), with increasing concentration as the menstrual cycle progressed from the follicular to the luteal phase. On the other hand, IL-1 and IL-6 levels did not vary throughout the menstrual cycle. Increased TNF-alpha was found in patients with pelvic adhesions compared with those with normal pelvis; the concentration of TNF-alpha was highest in mild compared with severe adhesions, but IL-1 concentration was elevated in the presence of severe adhesions. IL-6 levels were appreciably correlated with the grade of endometriosis ($P < 0.05$), but no significant correlations of either TNF-alpha or IL-1 concentrations were noted with the various grades of endometriosis. Although the precise role of TNF-alpha and IL-1 in adhesion formation is still unclear the results of this study signify that their concentration in the peritoneal fluid is associated with the degree of adhesions present [63].

A study correlating concentrations of mediators in serial samples of peritoneal fluid collected at diagnostic laparoscopy in one group, and at laparoscopy during the first 48 hours after laparoscopic adhesiolysis in a second group, found that the MMP-9 concentration was lower in the follicular phase than the luteal phase of the menstrual cycle. MMP-9 concentration was significantly less in women with pelvic adhesions than in women with a normal pelvis. The MMP-9/TIMP-1 ratio was significantly higher in women with considerable adhesions at second-look laparoscopy compared to women with minimal or no adhesions. The components of extracellular matrix remodeling may play an important part in the adhesion formation/reformation process [64].

Bloody peritoneal fluid (PF) is frequently present in the culde-sac of endometriosis patients and contains an array of biologically active factors. Iwabe T, et al2005 [65], recorded that the concentrations of tumor necrosis factor alpha (TNF-alpha) and interleukin-6 (IL-6) in PF from patients with endometriosis were considerably more elevated than that of patients with endometriosis. There were appreciably positive correlations between the levels of TNF-alpha and IL-6, which also correlated with the number and extent of red color peritoneal endometriosis. TNF-alpha enhanced the expression of IL-6 messenger RNA and protein in endometriotic stromal cells derived from chocolate cyst in a dose-dependent manner [66].

The involvement of T cells in the pathogenesis of endometriosis is a contentious matter. With the aim of investigating the role of T-cell implication in the pathogenesis of endometriosis. Szyllo K et al 2003 [67], conducted a study enrolling women aged 24-46 years with established diagnosis of endometriosis.All the patients studied underwent diagnostic laparoscopy.The distribution of T-lymphocyte subpopulations in peripheral blood (PB), peritoneal fluid (PF) and in endometriotic tissues (ET),as well as cytokines [interleukin (IL)-2, IL-4, IL-10, IL-12, interferon(IFN)-gamma] production by peripheral blood lymphocytes. IFN-gamma, tumor necrosis factor (TNF)-alpha, IL-4 and IL-6 was investigated..The experiments were done before and after 6months treatment with the GnRH-Analogous Goserelin.

Comparison of the lymphocyte subset re-distribution with regard to the American Fertility Society (AFS) stages and scores, showed no differences.. The significant increase in CD4:CD8 ratio, the decrease in the numberof natural killer (NK) cells in PB and the decrease in CD4:CD8 ratio in PF and ETof women with endometriosis was noted. The diminished IFN-gamma secretion by phytohemagglutinim (PHA)-stimulated lymphocytes in vitro derived from women with endometriosis and increased IL-4 production may be the cause of defective immunosurveillance against overgrowth of endometriotic tissues. The diminished NKcells number in PB of women with endometriosis supports such a hypothesis. The increased deposits of proinflammatory IL-6 and TNF-alpha in the T lymphocytes of women with endometriosis may be linked to T-regulatory lymphocyte function and their inability to suppress cell proliferation in endometriosis. GnRH-Analogous Goserelin treatment normalises cytokine production and improves patient recovery. The important functional and phenotypic differences between the lymphocytes from healthy women and women with endometriosis were noted. The diminished IFN-gamma production in relation to reduced NK cells number and the enhanced IL-4 production prior to the treatment and normalisation after the treatment signifies the involvement of the deregulated T-cell system in the growth stimulation and recruitment of endometriotic cells. The increased CD4:CD8 ratio, IL-6, TNF-alpha deposits and diminished anti-inflammatory IL-10 production by lymphocytes may have a role in the pathogenesis of endometriosis, and may secondarily impact the monocyte/macrophage function [67].

Genetic Aspect of Endometriosis:

There is mounting evidence in favour of a genetic basis for endometriosis. Endometriosis is most likely a complex trait, signifying that the disease is the outcome of an interaction between multiple genes and environment. As this condition does not have an obvious Mendelian pattern of inheritance and multiple gene loci confer vulnerability to the condition and interact with each other and the environment [68].

In a study [69] to illustrate the incidence of endometriosis in monozygotic twins. Twins were enrolled via the American Endometriosis Association and the National Endometriosis Society of Great Britain and via British gynecologists. Fourteen twin pairs were concordant for endometriosis, and two were discordant. Nine pairs of twins had moderate-severe endometriosis. These findings add to the mounting body of evidence that suggests endometriosis has a genetic basis [69].

It is well recognized that endometriosis is a condition exhibiting heritable proclivities. Polygenic/multifactorial etiology appears more plausible than Mendelian inheritance. It has also been hypothesized that endometriosis is analogous to neoplasia thus implying it as a multistep phenomenon of clonal origin [70].

Family and twin studies have shown that heritability accounts for endometriosis development to an extent similar to other complex genetic diseases [71].

It is well recognized that daughters or sisters of patients with endometriosis are at higher risk of developing endometriosis themselves; for example, low progesterone levels may be genetic, and may contribute to a hormone imbalance. There is an about 10-fold increased incidence in women with an affected first-degree relative [72]. One study found that in female siblings of patients with endometriosis the relative risk of endometriosis is 5.7:1 versus a control population [73].

With a view to detect molecular differences in the endometrium of women with endometriosis in exploring the pathogenesis and for developing novel approaches for the treatment of the condition. Richard O. Burney et al 2007 [74], conducted global gene expression analysis of endometrium from women with and without moderate/severe stage endometriosis and compared the gene expression signatures in different phases of the menstrual cycle. The study comprised; a) the transcriptome analysis; b) Paralleled gene expression analysis of endometrial specimens; c) gene expression involved in DNA synthesis and cellular mitosis in endometriosis and D) Comparative gene expression analysis of progesterone-regulated genes. The study revealed molecular dysregulation of the proliferative-to-secretory shift in endometrium of women with endometriosis, improved cellular survival and continual expression of genes concerned with DNA synthesis and cellular mitosis at the site of endometriosis. Comparative gene expression analysis of progesterone-regulated genes in secretory phase endometrium established the observation of attenuated progesterone response. Moreover it identified remarkable candidate susceptibility genes that may be linked with endometriosis, including FOXO1A, MIG6, and CYP26A1. Collectively these findings provide a framework for further investigations on causality and mechanisms underlying attenuated progesterone response in endometrium of women with endometriosis [74].

In this context it is pertinent to refer to MicroRNAs

(miRNAs), small noncoding RNAs that regulate gene expression, have essential roles in biological processes, including cell differentiation and proliferation. They mostly function as gene silencers and direct either target messenger RNA (mRNA) degradation or translational suppression It is well known that endometrial cells and glands of the uterus go through cyclic changes under the control of the sex steroid hormones estradiol-17beta and progesterone .Expression of miRNAs in human endometrium has been established,and hence the need to explore the role of miRNAs in modulating the expression of hormonally induced genes prompted the study by Satu Kuokkanen et al 2010 [75] . They found simultaneous differential miRNA and mRNA expression profiles of endometrial cells in the late proliferative and midsecretory phases. It was observed that; 1)differentially expressed mRNAs exposed cell cycle regulation as the most notably enriched pathway in the late proliferative-phase endometrial epithelium ($P = 5.7 \times 10^{-15}$), and 2) the enhancement of WNT signaling pathway in the proliferative phase. There was expression of 12 miRNAs (*MIR29B, MIR29C, MIR30B, MIR30D, MIR31, MIR193A-3P, MIR203, MIR204, MIR200C, MIR210, MIR582-5P, and MIR345*) which were appreciably up-regulated in the midsecretory-phase and were predicted to target many cell cycle genes. The suppressor effect of miRNAs on their target mRNA expression was evident from the observed decrease of cyclins and cyclin-dependent kinases, and *E2F3* (a known target of *MIR210*). Thus, their data imply that miRNAs down-regulate the expression of some cell cycle genes in the secretory-phase endometrial epithelium, thus suppressing cell proliferation [75].

Endometriosis is associated with abnormal growth or turn-over of cells, however, the genetic changes involved still awaits further exploration. A study [76], reported that the occurrence of somatic chromosomal changes in severe/late stage endometriosis was studied in four cases of endometriosis .With the aid of alpha-satellite sequence-specific DNA probes for chromosomes

7, 8, 11, 12, 16, 17, and 18, simultaneous two- and three-color FISH were performed to estimate the frequency of monosomic, disomic, and trisomic cells in normal control and endometriotic tissue specimens. One of the endometriosis samples showed, an appreciably higher frequency of monosomy for chromosome 17 (14.8%, χ^2_4 = 53.3, $P < 0.0001$) and 16 (8.8%, χ^2_4 = 11.4, $P < 0.05$). In a second case there was an augmented proportion of cells with chromosome 11 trisomy (14.8%, χ^2_4 = 96.2, $P < 0.0001$) In the third case, a distinct colony of nuclei with chromosome 16 monosomy (14.1%, χ^2_4 = 21.39, $P < 0.005$). A study found Acquired chromosome-specific aneuploidy may be implicated in endometriosis, reflecting clonal expansion of chromosomally abnormal cells. That candidate tumor suppressor genes and oncogenes which have been mapped to chromosomes 11, 16, and 17 imply that deletion or gain of chromosomes has a part to play in the pathogenesis and/or progression of endometriosis [76].

Another study [77], reported a relation between endometriosis and chromosome 10q26, while another study [78], discovered an association with the 7p15.2 region. Admittedly numerous challenges pose problems to genetic investigations on endometriosis because of the diverse manifestations and various forms of endometriosis. The problem is further compounded by factors such as strong gene-environmental interactions that might interfere with approaches to identify genetic variants involved [79].

Both linkage analysis and association studies have been conducted to recognize genetic determinants for the disease. Results from the linkage scan of 1,176 families collected jointly between an Australian and a UK group highlighted an important linkage to a novel susceptibility locus on chromosome 10q26. Gene variants with impact on the disease predilection have been assumed to exist and several candidates have been proposed, but their effects are yet to be established. The major categories of candidate genes studied have been those concerned with detoxification processes, sex steroid biosynthesis and action, immune system regulation. Admittedly numerous challenges pose problems to genetic investigations on endometriosis because of the diverse manifestations and various forms of endometriosis. Genome-wide association studies that survey most of the genome for causal genetic variants provide the potential for future progress [79].

Recent molecular cytogenetic investigations on endometriotic tissue and endometriosis-derived cell line revealed new proof that acquired chromosome-specific changes may be related to endometriosis, perhaps implying clonal expansion of chromosomally abnormal cells. Molecular DNA studies on the role of loss of heterozygosity in endometriotic lesions has detected candidate tumour suppressor gene loci, including 5q, 6q, 9p, 11q and 22q, that may paticipate in the genesis of endometrioid ovarian cancers.from endometriotic implants . Mutations in the tumour suppressor *PTEN* gene in the endometrioid subtype of epithelial ovarian cancer further indicates that somatic genetic alterations reflect early modification changes in the benign endometriotic cells. It is possible that genetic factors impact individual proneness to endometriosis. There is sign of proof that heritable allelic differences in drug-metabolizing enzymes may have significant part in the pathogenesis of endometriosis [80].

An array of disorders, such as insulin-dependent diabetes mellitus (IDDM), systemic lupus erythematosus (SLE), and pre-eclampsia, , mucous membrane pemphigoid are linked to particular HLA types [81-82], which are regarded as an immune response-related genes.

In view of the lack of any proven connection between endometriosis and HLA antigens and failure of previous studies employing serological analysis to report a statistically significant link between endometriosis and HLA allotype frequency. Keisuke Ishii et al 2002 [83], investigated to detect the possible relation between endometriosis HLA allotype frequency. In their study noted that the prevalence of the HLA-DRB1*1403 allele was significantly greater in patients with endometriosis than in the general controls. They [83] observed that the prevalence of HLA-DQB1*0301 in the former group was 16.3% relative to 8.3% in the overall control group and 7.7% in the females of the control group. The frequency of the HLA-DQB1*0301 allele was appreciably greater in endometriosis patients compared with the general controls Association in the frequencies of DPB1 alleles between the patients and controls was hardly noticeable. Thus their study lends support to imply that HLA systems may be implicated in the aetiology of endometriosis [83].

Oxford Endometriosis Gene Study (OXEGENE) is designed to discover whether there is a genetic cause for endometriosis, and to identify susceptibility loci involved in the development of endometriosis using the linkage analysis. DNA from sisters with surgically confirmed r-AFS stage II-IV disease and their parents are being collected to perform a genome-wide screen. There were 571 Families, 886 patients and 65 collaborators involving this study until the time that this manuscript was in preparation.

Endometriosis is an intricate disorder that has long been recognized as presenting heritable tendencies, with recurrence risks of 5-7% for first-degree relatives. Familial and epidemiologic studies substantiate its genetic basis and the disorder is of polygenic/multifactorial inheritance. The current investigational challenge is to determine the number and location of causative genes. Recent advances in molecular technology make identification and elucidation of these genes now possible [84].

Two genetic associations with endometriosis have been reported: 1) Polymorphism in galactose-1-phosphate uridyl transferase (GALT); 2) Null mutation in Glutathione S-transferase M1 (GSTM1) [85-86]. Enzymes belonging to the glutathione S-transferase family are involved in the two stage of detoxification of 2,3,7,8-Tetraachlorodibenzo-p-Dioxin (Dioxin) which is a potential pollutant for endometriosis development [85-86]. It will be of much interest to refer to the controversies surrounding the glutathione S-transferases (GST) M1/T1-endometriosis association. In view of the debate a meta-analysis of the GSTM1/GSTT1 genetic association studies of endometriosis was performed [87]. This meta-analysis involved 14 GSTM1 studies with 1539 cases and 1805 controls and nine GSTT1 studies with 746 cases and 834 controls, respectively, and it showed considerable heterogeneities among studies. There was no evidence that women with GSTM1 null genotype have augmented risk of developing endometriosis as compared with women with other genotypes. For GSTT1, the risk associated with the null genotype is 29% higher than other genotypes. Nevertheless, the author has cautioned that even this approximation should be viewed with skepticism as regards its questionable statistical significance [87].

To explore a possible connection between endometriosis, Müllerian anomalies, and possession of the N314D allele of the gene for galactose-1-phosphate uridyl transferase (GALT), a study was conducted and it comprised 33 women with endometriosis. The patients were DNA tested for the N314D mutation of GALT. Compared with endometriosis cases without the N314D allele, those cases with the allele tended to have more advanced disease and a family history of endometriosis. This in fact throws some light on one of the causes of endometriosis, in turn due to Muelleriam obstruction. Thus they were led them to infer that endometriosis may arise due to defects of canalization of the cervix leading to cervical stenosis and retrograde menstruation. The relevance of the N314D mutation, via this model, may derive from an association between abnormalities of galactose metabolism and vaginal agenesis which represents a canalization defect of the vaginal plate of the Müllerian tubercle, the same structure which gives rise to the cervix [88].

An investigation by Mayumi Morizane et al 2004 [89] was performed to look at the frequency of glutathione S-transferase M1 and T1 (GSTM1 and GSTT1) null mutations in women with endometriosis in a Japanese population. The study enrolled one hundred fourteen unrelated women with endometriosis Samples of Umbilical cord blood samples from 179 female newborn infants served as population controls. Genomic DNA isolated from endometriosis patients and controls were subjected to multiple polymerase chain reactions to determine the GSTM1 and GSTT1 genotypes. There were no significant differences in the frequencies of the GSTM1 ($P = .83$, odds ratio 0.95) and GSTT1 ($P = .24$, odds ratio 0.75) null mutations between endometriosis patients and controls. Their findings do not support that the GSTM1 and GSTT1 null mutations are likely to be associated with an increased risk of endometriosis in a Japanese population [89].

Endometriosis is well established as a condition

showing heritable tendencies. Polygenic/multifactorial etiology appears far more likely to be the etiology than Mendelian inheritance. The current task is to determine the number and location of genes responsible for endometriosis. The revision should include the basis for concluding that endometriosis is a genetic disorder of polygenic/multifactorial inheritance and outline selected strategies for identifying the number and location of causative genes. It also exemplifies their approach to testing the hypothesis that endometriosis bears similarity to neoplasia and, thus, is a multistep phenomenon of clonal origin [70].

A few words of proteomics and its usefulness in the study endometriosis with new proteins that have a potential role in the initiation and progression of endometriosis: it also serves as stage or for more investigations on mechanisms implicated in the pathogenesis of endometriosis.

The detection of molecular differences in the endometrium of women with endometriosis is an essential in the right direction of exploring the pathogenesis of this condition and for developing new strategies for the treatment of the condition. Rai P, et al 2010 [90] studied protein expression analysis of eutopic endometrium from women with and without endometriosis it was observed that. it revealed molecular dysregulation of more than 70 proteins in the proliferative phase of eutopic endometrium in stage IV and secretory phase of stage II, III and IV endometriosis Mass spectrometry detected , 48 proteins spots which were consistently differentially expressed from stage II to IV endometriosis were identified. The differentially expressed proteins include structural proteins, proteins involved in stress response, protein-folding and protein-turnover, immunity, energy production, signal transduction, RNA biogenesis, protein biosynthesis, and nuclear proteins. Immunoblot and immunohistochemical analyses confirmed the observed changes in eight representative proteins. The present study provides identification of new players that have a potential role in the initiation and progression of endometriosis and also sets a framework for further investigations on mechanisms underlying the pathogenesis of endometriosis [90].

Familial clustering in Rhesus monkeys

Familial tendency of disease supporting the hypothesis that endometriosis has a genetic basis was discovered in these studies. The clinical features at surgery and histological characteristics of the disease in the rhesus monkey resemble those in human. Therefore, the clearer understanding of the epidemiology and inheritability of the disease may emerge from studying spontaneous endometriosis in rhesus monkey colonies (Macaca Mulatta). Oxford Group is collaborating with California Regional Primate Research Center (CRPRC) and Wisconsin Regional Primate Research Center (WRPRC) to study the epidemiology and inheritability of endometriosis. They have identified 121 (8.3%) affected rhesus monkeys among the autopsy records of the 1459 female animals that they died, aged 4 years of more, in the colony between 1982-1996 at CRPRC. They are trying to determine the familial tendency in these affected animals by analyzing the entire colony records over 9000 females from 1965-1977. Hadfield et al studied the autopsy records of 399 rhesus monkeys that died in the WRPRC colony between 1980 and 1995 and reported a prevalence rate of 20% in animals aged 4 years or older at death and 29% in animals aged 10 years or older at death [91].

The development of an animal model of endometriosis is vital for the study of disease pathogenesis and therapeutic intercession. These models will improve the methods of evaluation the causes for the subfertility associated with disease and offer the most important justification of treatment modulators. Presently rodents and non-human primate models have been developed, but each model has its own constraints They have summarized the recent findings and theories on the pathogenesis of endometriosis disease progression and the efficacy of therapeutic targets using the experimental induced model of endometriosis in the baboon (*Papio anubis*) [91].

The chicken chorioallantoic membrane (CAM) model can be regarded as an animal model in the broader sense. Although innovatively, it had been developed to study the invasive, metastatic and angiogenic potential of neoplastic cells [92]. It is now an established as a model for endometriosis by culturing fragments of human endometrial tissue on the basal layer of the CAM of fertilized chicken eggs after prior incubation for 7-10 days [93-94]. Endometrial fragments from the proliferative and secretory phase of the menstrual cycle as well as the menstrual endometrium invade across the epithelium into the mesenchymal layer and develop endometriosis-like lesions in this layer of the CAM within 3 days after grafting of the human tissue. It was shown that these endometrial fragments needed to contain intact glandular structures as well as stromal components [92-94].

Stem cell theory of endometriosis:

Adult stem cells are thought to be responsible for the high regenerative capacity of the human endometrium, and have been implicated in the pathology of endometriosis and endometrial carcinoma. The RNA-binding protein Musashi-1 is associated with maintenance and asymmetric cell division of neural and epithelial progenitor cells. Götte, M.et al 2008 [95], investigated expression and localization of Musashi-1 in endometrial, endometrio tic and endometrial carcinoma tissue specimens of 46 patients. qPCR revealed significantly increased *Musashi-1* mRNA expression in the endometrium compared to the myometrium. Musashi-1 protein expression presented as nuclear or cytoplasmic immunohistochemical staining of single cells in endometrial glands, and of single cells and cell groups in the endometrial stroma. Immunofluorescence microscopy revealed colocalization of Musashi-1 with its molecular target Notch-1 and telomerase. In proliferative endometrium, the proportion of Musashi-1-positive cells in the basalis layer was significantly increased 1.5-fold in the stroma, and three-fold in endometrial glands compared to the functionalis. The number of Musashi-1 expressing cell groups was significantly increased (four-fold) in proliferative compared to secretory endometrium. Musashi-1 expressing stromal cell and cell group numbers were significantly increased (five-fold) in both endometriotic and endometrial carcinoma tissue compared to secretory endometrium. A weak to moderate, diffuse cytoplasmic glandular staining was seen in 50% of the endometriosis cases and in 75% of the endometrioid carcinomas compared to complete absence in normal endometrial samples. Their findings highlight the importance the role of Musashi-1-expressing endometrial progenitor cells in proliferating endometrium, endometriosis and endometrioid uterine carcinoma, and uphold the perception of a stem cell origin of endometriosis and endometrial carcinoma [95].

A retrospective analysis on necropsy records from a rhesus monkey colony of 66 monkeys with histologically verified endometriosis and 248 control subjects. to assess the age-related incidence of endometriosis revealed that the incidence of endometriosis increases progressively across the life span, eventually affecting 21-45% of aged monkeys over 20 years of age [96].

While it is common to see endometriosis in humans it has also been observed in animals. This is evident from studies that follow. An observational longitudinal study was conducted by D'Hooghe TM, et al [97], at the Institute of Primate Research, Nairobi (Kenya), using 24 baboons with laparoscopically confirmed normal pelves underwent 67 serial laparoscopies for a variable length of follow-up,from one month to 32 months. Considering the variable length of follow-up, they used life-table analysis to calculate the cumulative incidence of endometriosis. The cumulative incidence of minimal endometriosis (proven by histology) was 64% up to 32 months of follow-up. The eight baboons that developed confirmed endometriosis were followed over longer periods of time and had undergone more laparoscopies than the animals that did not develop the condition. Their studies concluded that there is a high incidence of minimal endometriosis in baboons, which increases with the duration of follow-up and the number of repeat laparoscopies [97].

Sherry E. Rier et al 1993 [98], determined the incidence of endometriosis in a colony of rhesus monkeys constantly exposed to 2,3,7,8-tetrachlorodibenzo-p-dioxin (TCDD or dioxin) for 4 years. Ten years after cessation of dioxin treatment, endometriosis was diagnosed at laparoscopy and the severity of disease was assessed. The incidence of endometriosis was directly correlated with dioxin exposure and the severity of disease was dependent upon the dose administered ($p < 0.001$). Three of 7 animals exposed to 5 ppt dioxin (43%) and 5 of 7 animals exposed to 25 ppt dioxin (71%) had moderate to severe endometriosis. In contrast, the frequency of disease in the control group was 33%, similar to an overall prevalence of 30% in 304 rhesus monkeys with no dioxin exposure. This 15-year study implies that latent female reproductive abnormalities may be associated with dioxin exposure in the rhesus [98].

Environmental factors

Our body works it's best to cope with hundreds of synthetic chemicals every day, if anything goes wrong during this process, free radicals form as well as increasing the risk of some of the cells of the peritoneum to develop into endometrial cells.

Studies have provided important information about environmental factors and their potential influence on development of endometriosis [99]. For example, rhesus monkeys exposed to whole-body proton irradiation have a higher frequency of endometriosis than controls (53% *vs* 26%) [100]. Also, rhesus monkeys exposed to 5-25 ppm dioxin per day for 4 years developed endometriosis that was dose-dependent in staging [99-101].

Extrapolation to women was initially thought to be epidemiologically plausible, especially with the publication of a report that Belgium, with the highest dioxin pollution in the world, has the highest incidence of endometriosis as well as the highest prevalence of severe endometriosis [102]. However, two subsequent prospective studies from Italy and Belgium found no significantly increased risk of endometriosis in women who have been exposed to dioxin [99, 103-104].

To date, there has been no epidemiological study definitively linking one class of chemicals to the risk of endometriosis, although oestrogen-like compounds in the environment have been suggested [105]. The lack of a definitive link is not surprising because people are exposed to a multiplicity of chemicals, with mechanisms of action that might vary with dose, timing of exposure (in utero, childhood, peripubertally, adult), route of exposure, and synergy with other chemicals, [105] all proceeding against unique genetic backgrounds [99].

A survey by the Centers for Disease Control and Prevention (National Report on Human Exposure to Environmental Chemicals) is now under way; biomonitoring of 145 chemicals in 2500 people in the USA is carried out every 2 years [99]. A major challenge is to relate the data to disease risk. Although biomonitoring for specific chemicals could be interesting, the effect on health, including the development of endometriosis, will probably take years to elucidate, if there is indeed causality. Recent reviews underscore the roles of the toxic chemicals, lifestyle, and reproductive health; [99, 106-107].

Few studies that have been undertaken suggest that lifestyle and dietary factors may be associated with susceptibility to developing endometriosis [108-110]. The results of these epidemiological studies found that a diet high in fruit and vegetables and low in meat products was protective against developing endometriosis. Additionally, women with few or no children and low body mass index (BMI) were at a higher risk of developing endometriosis.

Other authors have suggested that exposure to synthetic compounds such as dioxin and other polychlorinated biphenyls (PCBs) could lead to the development of endometriosis due to their effects as endocrine disruptors [112-113] Dioxin is a by-product of the chlorine bleaching process used in the wood pulp processing industry, this also includes the manufacture of tampons which is thought to be a major source of dioxin exposure in women. However, the associations with dioxin are mainly based on animal data [114-116], which some authors criticise for poor study design and data analysis [117] Human data on dioxin exposure and endometriosis risk is scant and in some cases appear contradictory. For example, a study reported that the incidence of deeply infiltrating endometriosis in Belgium, reportedly the highest in the world, correlates with high dioxin exposure through breast milk [118]. However, another study assessed massive dioxin exposure from the Seveso incident in Italy during the summer of 1976, whereby a chemical manufacturing plant accidentally released 1Kg of dioxin into the atmosphere, showering the neighbouring residential areas with dioxin. Although extremely high levels of dioxin contamination were found in soil and water samples, no significant increase in endometriosis incidence were observed, even after a 26 year follow up study [119] Despite reported increased serum dioxin levels [120-121] and increased serum levels of bisphenols [121] observed in endometriosis patients, a conclusive association between environmental toxicant exposure and increased risk of developing endometriosis has yet to be established. Given the variety and conflicting notions pertaining to the origin and development of endometriosis, it becomes clear why endometriosis is often referred to as the *'disease of theories'* [122].

Xenoestrogen overload: Xenoestrogens are but environmental chemicals with estrogenic activity [123]. Xenohormones are new, and have only been known in since about 1991. They are by-products of manufacturing processes, such as synthetic chemicals, which simulate the effect of natural estrogen produced by our body. Some of these Xenoestrogens like DDE (a metabolite of DDT) may persist in the body fat for decades. Many of these mimicking hormones which were once thought to occur in pesticides were regarded as inert materials. Xenoestrogens,have attracted considerable attention theoretically agreement is centred around the fact that such compounds, in high doses, may induce developmental, reproductive and tumorigenic effects together with a critical appraisal of methods to detect and quantitate the estrogenic activity of synthetic and naturally occurring chemicals [123].

The manner in which Xenoestrogens are implicated in the etiology of endometriosis.is briefly described below. During the rush of estrogen at the commencement of menstrual cycle, over-production of xenoestrogen induces hormone imbalance leading to over-stimulation of certain hormones, inducing metaplasia of peritoneal lining cells into endometrial cells.
Overdose of Environmental toxins from food air, or contact through skin cause hormonal imbalance leading to xenoestrogens enhancing the risk of endometriosis. In addition Xenoestrogens being toxic tend to weaken the immune system Overdose of xenoestrogens not only disturbs the production of natural estrogen from our body, but it also predisposes to the generation of free radicals and weakens the immune system to defend against any bacteria and virus as well as implanting endometrial cells in unusual sites in the body. Again overload of xenoestrogen through food consumption may stimulate high level of estrogen production leading to hormone imbalance as well as augmenting the risk of endometriosis. According to the coelomic metaplasia theory Xenoestrogens toxify and disrupt the normal cell development favouring the risk of some of the peritoneal

cells to develop into endometrial cells. Finally Xenoestrogens by augmenting the production of estrogen induce hormone imbalance resulting in disruption of menstrual cycle promoting the development of growth of endometriosis. Endometriosis as is well known is an estrogen-dependent disease, c-fos is an early transcription factor that has been documented to be linked to estradiol-dependent cell proliferation. Morsch DM et al 2009 [124], performed a study to assess the c-fos gene and protein expression in pelvic endometriotic implants in comparison to normal endometrium from infertile women. This open, prospective and controlled study comprising 15 infertile women with endometriosis and 19 control infertile women. Endometrial and endometriotic biopsies were performed at the follicular phase and the samples were processed for RT-PCR and immunohistochemistry.). c-fos gene expression was more elevated in endometriotic implants (1.32 +/- 0.13; P = 0.011) than in eutopic endometrium from patients with endometriosis (0.97 +/- 0.11) or from the control group (0.91 +/- 0.05). Besides, immunohistochemistry revealed a more copious distribution of c-Fos in the stroma of endometriotic tissue relative to eutopic endometrium. These findings imply the role of c-fos may in the molecular mechanisms of estrogen action on the initiation and evolution of endometriosis [124].

Xenoestrogen bisphenol A (BPA) simulates estrogen both in vivo and in vitro. One of the explicit objectives of the study by R Steinmetz,et al 1998 [125], was to characterize the short term effects of BPA on cell proliferation and c-fos expression in the uterus and vagina, Treatment with single high doses of BPA induced cell proliferation in the uterus and vagina of ovariectomized F344 rats. By quantitative RT-PCR it was shown that both BPA and E2 increased c-fos messenger RNA levels in the uterus 14- to 16-fold within 2 h, which returned to basal levels after 6 h [123]. It is relevant at this juncture to refer to the studies of Morsch DM, et al 2009 [124] which imply the role of c-fos may in the molecular mechanisms of estrogen action on the initiation and evolution of endometriosis.

The immune system which is under composite control can react promptly to the environment, recent findings emphasize the likely implication of environmental xenobiotic chemicals which can alter normal immune function. Currently much attention is focused on chemicals which influence sex steroids in the genesis of immune diseases; this stems from the increased occurrence of autoimmune disease in women, the gender variation in the immune response, as well as the immunomodulatory influence of sex steroids, Furthermore, recent reports indicate that certain environmental chemicals can exert their influence on nuclear hormone receptors, besides sex hormone receptors, and affectt immune reactions [124].

References

1. Seli E, Berkkanoglu Arici AM. Pathogenesis of endometriosis. Obstetrics and Gynecology Clinics of North America 2003; 30(1):41-61.

2. Oral, E. & Arici, A.. Pathogenesis of endometriosis. Obstetric and Gynecology Clinics 1997; 24 (2): 219-233.

3. Matsuura, K., Ohtake, H., Katabuchi, H. & Okamura, H. Coelomic Metaplasia Theory of Endometriosis: Evidence from in Vivo Studies and an in vitro experimental Model. Gynecologic and Obstetric Investigation 1999; 47 (Suppl1): 18-22.

4. Sampson JA. Ovarian hematomas of endometrial type (perforating hemorrhagic cysts of the ovary) and implantation adenomas of endometrial type. Boston Med Surg J 1922; 186: 445-73.

5. Sampson JA. Peritoneal endometriosis due to menstrual dissemination of endometrial tissue into the peritoneal cavity. Am J Obst Gynecol 1927; 14: 442-69.

6. Vinatier, D., Cosson, M. & Dufour, P. Is endometriosis an endometrial disease? European Journal of Obstetrics, Gynaecology and Reproductive Biology 2000; 91(2): 113-25.

7. Keetle, WC. & Stein, RJ. The viability of the cast off menstrual endometrium. American Journal of Obstetrics and Gynecology 1951; 61: 440.

8. Kale, S., Shuster, M. & Sahmgold, I. Endometrioma in a caesarean scar: case report and review of literature. American Journal of Obstetrics and Gynecology 1971; 111: 596.

9. Scott RB, Te Linde RW, Wharton LR Jr. Further studies on experimental endometriosis. Am J Obstet Gynecol. 1953; 66:1082.

10. Liu DT, Hitchcock A. Endometriosis: its association with retrograde menstruation, dysmenorrhoea and tubal pathology. Br J Obstet Gynaecol. Aug 1986; 93(8):859-62.

11. Kruitwagen RF, Poels LG, Willemsen WN, de Ronde IJ, Jap PH, Rolland R. Endometrial epithelial cells in peritoneal fluid during the early follicular phase. Fertil Steril. Feb 1991; 55(2):297-303.

12. D'Hooghe TM, Bambra CS, Raeymaekers BM, Koninckx PR. Increased prevalence and recurrence of retrograde menstruation in baboons with spontaneous endometriosis. *Hum Reprod*. Sep 1996; 11(9):2022-5.

13. Thomas M. D'Hooghe, Charanjit S, Barbara M. Raeymaekers, Inge De Jonge, Jo M. Lauweryns and P. R. Koninckx. Intrapelvic injection of menstrual endometrium causes endometriosis in baboons (Papio cynocephalus and Papio Anubis). American Journal of Obstetrics and Gynecology 1995; 173(1): 125-134.

14. Wu MY, Ho HN. The role of cytokines in endometriosis. Am J Reprod Immunol 2003; 49(5):285-96.

15. Osamu Yoshino, Yutaka Osuga, Kaori Koga, Yasushi Hirota, Tetsuya Hirata, Xie Ruimeng, Li Na, Tetsu Yano, Osamu Tsutsum, Yuji Taketani. FR 167653, a p38 mitogen-activated protein kinase inhibitor, suppresses the development of endometriosis in a murine model. Journal of Reproductive Immunology 2006; 72(1-2): 85-93.

16. Philippe R. Koninckz, Anastasia Ussia. Epidemiology of endometriosis. Book chapter written April 2003; 5: 1-16.

17. Redwine D. Was Sampson wrong? Fertil.Steril.

2002;78:686.

18. Koninckx PR, Barlow D, Kennedy S. Implantation versus infiltration: the Sampson versus the endometriotic disease theory. Gynecol. Obstet.Invest 1999;47 Suppl 1:3-9.

19. Halme J, Hammond MG, Hulka JF, Raj SG, Talbert LM. Retrograde menstruation in healthy women and in patients with endometriosis. Obstet Gynecol 1984; 64:151-154.

20. Kitawaki J, Kado N, Ishihara H, Koshiba H, Kitaoka Y, Honjo H. Endometriosis: the pathophysiology as an estrogen-dependent disease. J Steroid Biochem Mol Biol. 2002; 83(1-5):149-55.

21. Serdar E. Bulun, Zongjuan Fang, Gonca Imir, Bilgin Gurates, Mitsutoshi Tamura, Bertan Yilmaz, David Langoi, Sanober Amin, Sijun Yang and Santanu Deb. Aromatase in endometriosis Semin Reprod Med. 2004; 22(1):

22. Noble LS, Simpson ER, Johns A, Bulun SE. Aromatase expression in endometriosis. J Clin Endocrinol Metab 1996; 81:174-179

23. Bulun SE, Simpson ER, Word RA. Expression of the CYP19 gene and its product aromatase cytochrome P450 in human leiomyoma tissues and cells in culture. J Clin Endocrinol Metab 1994; 78:736-743

24. Noble LS, Takayama K, Zeitoun KM, et al. Prostaglandin E_2 stimulates aromatase expression in endometriosis-derived stromal cells. J Clin Endocrinol Metab 1997; 82:600-606.

25. Michael MD, Michael LF, Simpson ER. A CRE-like sequence that binds CREB and contributes to cAMP-dependent regulation of the proximal promoter of the human aromatase P450 (CYP19) gene. Mol Cell

Endocrinol 1997; 134:147-156.

26. Michael MD, Kilgore MW, Morohashi KI, Simpson ER. Ad4BP/SF-1 regulates cyclic AMP-induced transcription from the proximal promoter (PII) of the human aromatase P450 (CYP19) gene in the ovary. J Biol Chem 1995; 270:13561-13566.

27. Ackerman GE, Smith ME, Mendelson CR, MacDonald PC, Simpson ER. Aromatization of androstenedione by human adipose tissue stromal cells in monolayer culture. J Clin Endocrinol Metab 1981;53:412-417

28. MacDonald PC, Rombaut RP, Siiteri PK. Plasma precursors of estrogen, I: Extent of conversion of plasma Δ^4-androstenedione to estrone in normal males and non-pregnant normal, castrate and adrenalectomized females. J Clin Endocrinol Metab 1967;27:1103-1111

29. MacDonald PC, Edman CD, Hemsell DL, Porter JC, Siiteri PK. Effect of obesity on conversion of plasma androstenedione to estrone in postmenopausal women with and without endometrial cancer. Am J Obstet Gynecol 1978;130:448-455

30. Simpson ER, Mahendroo MS, Means GD, et al. Aromatase cytochrome P450, the enzyme responsible for estrogen biosynthesis. Endocr Rev 1994;15:342-355

31. Noble LS, Simpson ER, Johns A, Bulun SE. Aromatase expression in endometriosis. J Clin Endocrinol Metab 1996; 81:174-179

32. Zeitoun K, Takayama K, Michael MD, Bulun SE. Stimulation of aromatase P450 promoter (II) activity in endometriosis and its inhibition in endometrium are regulated by competitive binding of SF-1 and COUP-TF to the same cis-acting element. Mol Endocrinol 1999;13:239-253

33. Noble LS, Takayama K, Zeitoun KM, et al.

Prostaglandin E_2 stimulates aromatase expression in endometriosis-derived stromal cells. J Clin Endocrinol Metab 1997;82:600-606

34. Tamura M, Deb S, Sebastian S, Okamura K, Bulun SE. Estrogen up-regulates cyclooxygenase-2 via estrogen receptor in human uterine microvascular endothelial cells. Fertil Steril 2004. In press.

35. Khorram O, Taylor RN, Ryan IP, Schall TJ, Landers DV. Peritoneal fluid concentrations of the cytokine RANTES correlate with the severity of endometriosis. Am J Obstet Gynecol 1993;169:1545-1549

36. Sharpe-Timms KL, Penney LL, Zimmer RL, Wright JA, Zhang Y, Surewicz K. Partial purification and amino acid sequence analysis of endometriosis protein-II (ENDO-II) reveals homology with tissue inhibitor of metalloproteinases-1 (TIMP-1). J Clin Endocrinol Metab 1995;80:3784-3787.

37. Hill JA. Immunology and endometriosis. Fertil Steril 1992; 58:262-264

38. Kitawaki J, Kado N, Ishihara H, Koshiba H, Kitaoka Y, Honjo H. Endometriosis: the pathophysiology as an estrogen-dependent disease. J Steroid Biochem Mol Biol. 2002; 83(1-5):149-55.

39. Salem ML. Estrogen, a double-edged sword: modulation of TH1- and TH2-mediated inflammations by differential regulation of TH1/TH2 cytokine production. Curr Drug Targets Inflamm Allergy. 2004 Mar;3(1):97-104.

40. Verena Mönckedieck, Carolin Sannecke, Bettina Husen, Michael Kumbartsk Rainer Kimmig, Martin Tötsch, Elke Winterhagerd Ruth Grümmer. Progestins inhibit expression of MMPs and of angiogenic factors in human ectopic endometrial lesions in a mouse model Mol. Hum. Reprod 2009; 15(10): 633-643.

41. J. Szamatowicz, P. Laudański, and I. Tomaszewska. Matrix metalloproteinase-9 and tissue inhibitor of matrix metalloproteinase-1: a possible role in the pathogenesis of endometriosis Hum. Reprod 2002; 17 (2): 284-288.

42. Seli E. Endometriosis: interaction of immune and endocrine systems. Semin Reprod Med. 2003; 21(2):135-44.

43. Batt RE, Smith RA, Buck Louis GM, Martin DC, Chapron C, Koninckx PR, Yeh J. Müllerianosis. Histol Histopathol. 2007; 22(10):1161-6.

44. Batt RE, Smith RA, Buck GM, Severino MF, Naples JD. Müllerianosis Prog Clin Biol Res 1990; 323:413-26.

45. Schenken RS, Johnson JV, Riehl RM. c-myc protooncogene polypeptide expression in endometriosis. Am J Obstet Gynecol. 1991; 164(4):1031-6;

46. May K, Becker CM. Endometriosis and angiogenesis. Minerva Ginecol. 2008; 60(3):24.

47. Matsuura K, Ohtake H, Katabuchi H, Okamura H. Coelomic metaplasia theory of endometriosis: evidence from in vivo studies and an in vitro experimental model. Gynecol Obstet Invest. 1999; 47 Suppl 1:18-20.

48. I. Velasco ruiz, A. Campos Ferrer, P. Acién Alvarez, F. Quereda seguí. Antiendometrial antibodies and endometriosis. Obestet Gynecol 1990; 75(6):914-8.

49. Mathur S, Garza DE, Smith LF. Endometrial autoantigens eliciting immunoglobulin IgG, IgA, and IgM responses in endometriosis. Fertil Steril. 1990; 54(1):56-63.

50. Pillai S, Zhou GX, Arnaud P, Jiang H, Butler WJ, Zhang H. Antibodies to endometrial transferrin and alpha 2-Heremans Schmidt (HS) glycoprotein in patients with endometriosis. Am J Reprod Immunol 1996; 35(5):483-94.

51. D'Cruz OJ, Wild RA, Haas GG Jr, Reichlin M. Antibodies to carbonic anhydrase in endometriosis: prevalence, specificity, and relationship to clinical and laboratory parameters. Fertil Steril 1996; 66(4):547-56.

52. Sundqvist J., Falconer H., Seddighzadeh M., Vodolazkaia A., Fassbender A., Kyama C., Bokor A., Stephansson O., Padyukov L., Gemzell-Danielsson K., D'Hooghe T.M. Endometriosis and autoimmune disease: association of susceptibility to moderate/severe endometriosis with CCL21 and HLA-DRB1. Fertil. Steril. 2011; 95:437-440.

53. Rasheed K, Atta H, Taha TF, Azmy O, Sabry D, Selim M, El-Sawaf A, Bibars M, Ramzy A, El-Garf W, Anwar JSRM Vol VI Issue: 3.

54. Dmowski WP, Gebel HM, Braun DP. The role of cell-mediated immunity in pathogenesis of endometriosis. Am J Reprod Immunol. 1996; 35(2):118-22.

55. Chi-Chen Chang, Yao-Yuan Hsieh, Fuu-Jen Tsai, Chang-Hai Tsai, Horng-Der Tsai, Cheng-Chieh Lin. The proline form of p53 codon 72 polymorphism is associated with endometriosis. Fertility and Sterility 2002; 77(1): 43-45.

56. Vercellini P, Trecca D, Oldani S, Fracchiolla NS, Neri A, Crosignani PG. Analysis of p53 and ras gene mutations in endometriosis. Gynecol Obstet Invest 1994; 38:70-1.

57. Sakamoto T, Repasky WT, Uchida K, Hirata A, Hirata F. Modulation of cell death pathways to apoptosis and necrosis of H2O2-treated rat thymocytes by lipocortin I. Biochem Biophys Res Commun 1996; 220: 643-647.

58. Chun-yan, LANG Jing-he, LIU Hai-yuan and ZHOU Hui-mei. Expression of Annexin-1 in patients with endometriosis. Chinese Medical Journal 2008; 121(10):927-931.

59. Radke S, Austermann J, Russo-Marie F, Gerke V,

Rescher U. Specific association of annexin 1 with plasma membrane-resident and internalized EGF receptors mediated through the protein core domain. FEBS Lett 2004; 578 (1-2): 95-98.

60. Skouteris GG, Schröder CH. The hepatocyte growth factor receptor kinase-mediated phosphorylation of lipocortin-1 transduces the proliferating signal of the hepatocyte growth factor. J Biol Chem 1996; 271: 27266-27273.

61. Varticovski L, Chahwala SB, Whitman M, Cantley L, Schindler D, Chow EP, et al. Location of sites in human lipocortin I that are phosphorylated by protein tyrosine kinases and protein kinases A and C. Biochemistry 1988; 27: 3682-3690.

62. Dmowski WP. Immunological aspects of endometriosis. Int J Gynaecol Obstet 1995; 50 (Suppl 1): S3-S10.

63. Cheong YC, Shelton JB, Laird SM, Richmond M, Kudesia G, Li TC, Ledger WL. IL-1, IL-6 and TNF-alpha concentrations in the peritoneal fluid of women with pelvic adhesions. Hum Reprod. 2002; 17(1): 69-75.

64. Cheong YC, Shelton JB, Laird SM, Li TC, Ledger WL, Cooke ID. Peritoneal fluid concentrations of matrix metalloproteinase-9, tissue inhibitor of metalloproteinase-1, and transforming growth factor-beta in women with pelvic adhesions. Fertil Steril 2003; 79(5): 1168-75.

65. Iwabe T, Harada T, Terakawa N. Role of cytokines in endometriosis-associated infertility. Gynecol Obstet Invest. 2002; 53 Suppl 1:19-25.

66. Hammond MG, Oh ST, Anners J, Surrey ES, Halme J. The effect of growth factors on the proliferation of human endometrial stromal cells in culture. Am J Obstet Gynecol 1993; 168:1131-6.

67. Szyllo K, Tchorzewski H, Banasik M, Glowacka E,

Lewkowicz P, Kamer-Bartosinska The involvement of T lymphocytes in the pathogenesis of endometriotic tissues overgrowth in women with endometriosis. Mediators Inflamm. 2003; 12(3):131-8.

68. Erkut Attar,. Current Concepts and Research in the Pathogenesis of Endometriosis. http://www.endometriosiszone.org. Accessed 19th March 2014.

69. Hadfield RM, Mardon HJ, Barlow DH, Kennedy SH. Endometriosis in monozygotic twins.Fertil Steril. 1997 Nov;68(5):941-2.

70. Simpson JL, Bischoff FZ. Heritability and molecular genetic studies of endometriosis. Ann N Y Acad Sci. 2002; 955:239-51.

71. Vigano P, Somigliana E, Vignali M, Busacca M, Blasio AM. Genetics of endometriosis: current status and prospects. Front Biosci. 2007; 12:3247-55.

72. Dharmesh Kapoor and Willy Davila. 'Endometriosis', eMedicine (2005).

73. Kashima K, Ishimaru T, Okamura H, et al. Familial risk among Japanese patients with endometriosis. International Journal of Gynaecology and Obstetrics 2004; 84 (1): 61–4.

74. Richard O. Burney, Said Talbi, Amy E. Hamilton, Kim Chi Vo, Mette Nyegaard, Camran R. Nezhat, Bruce A. Lessey and Linda C. Giudice 2007 Gene Expression Analysis of Endometrium Reveals Progesterone Resistance and Candidate Susceptibility Genes in Women with Endometriosis. Endocrinology 2007; 148(8): 3814-3826.

75.Satu Kuokkanen, Bo Chen, Laureen Ojalvo, Lumie Benard, Nanette Santoro, and Jeffrey W. Pollard. Genomic Profiling of MicroRNAs and Messenger RNAs

Reveals Hormonal Regulation in MicroRNA Expression in Human Endometrium1 Biology of Reproduction 2010; 82(4): 791-801.

76. Jong-Chul Shin, Helen L. Ross, Sherman Elias, Dianne D. Nguyen, Dorothy Mitchell-Leef, Joe Leigh Simpson and F. Z. Bischoff. Detection of chromosomal aneuploidy in endometriosis by multi-color fluorescence in situ hybridization (FISH Human Genetics 1997; 100 (3-4): 401-406.

77. Treloar SA, Wicks J, Nyholt DR, et al. Genomewide linkage study in 1,176 affected sister pair families identifies a significant susceptibility locus for endometriosis on chromosome 10q26. American Journal of Human Genetics 2005; 77 (3): 365–76.

78. Painter JN et al. "Genome-wide association study identifies a locus at 7p15.2 associated with endometriosis". Nature Genetics 2010; 43 (1): 51–54.

79. Vigano P, Somigliana E, Vignali M, Busacca M, Blasio AM. Genetics of endometriosis: current status and prospects. Front Biosci. 2007; 12:3247-55.

80. Farideh Z. Bischoff, and Joe Leigh Simpson. Heritability and molecular genetic studies of endometriosis. Hum. Reprod. Update 2000; 6 (1): 37-44.

81. Setterfield, J., Theron, J., Vaughan, R., Welsh, K., Mallon, E., Wojnarowska, F., Challacombe, S. and Black, M. (2001), Mucous membrane pemphigoid: HLA-DQB1*0301 is associated with all clinical sites of involvement and may be linked to antibasement membrane IgG production. British Journal of Dermatology 2001; 145: 406–414.

82. F Pociot, and M F McDermott. Genetics of type 1 diabetes mellitus Genes and Immunity. 2002;3: 235–249.

83. **Keisuke Ishii, Koichi Takakuwa, Takuya Mitsui** and **Kenichi Tanaka**. Studies on the human leukocyte antigen-DR in patients with endometriosis: genotyping of HLA-DRB1 alleles. Hum. Reprod 2002; 17 (3): 560-563.

84. Bischoff F, Simpson JL. Genetic basis of endometriosis. Ann N Y Acad Sci. 2004;1034: 284-99.

85. Baranova H., Botorishvilli R., Canis M., et al. Glutathioe S-transferase M1 gene polymorphism and susceptibility to endometriosis in a French population. Mol Hum Reprod 1997; 3:775-80.

86. Baranov V.S., Ivaschenko T., Bakay B.., et al. Proportion of the GSTM1 0/0 phenotype in some Slavic populations and its correlation with cystic fibrosis and some multifactorial diseases. Hum Genet 1996; 97:516-20).

87. Sun-Wei Guo. Glutathione S-transferases M1/T1 gene polymorphisms and endometriosis: a meta-analysis of genetic association studies Mol. Hum. Reprod 2005;11 (10): 729-743.

88. Cramer DW, Hornstein MD, Ng WG, Barbieri RL. Endometriosis associated with the N314D mutation of galactose-1-phosphate uridyl transferase (GALT). Mol Hum Reprod. 1996; 2(3):149-52.

89. Mayumi Morizane, Shigeki Yoshida, Satoshi Nakago, Shinya HamanaTakeshi Maruo, Stephen Kennedy, No Association of Endometriosis With Glutathione S-Transferase M1 and T1 Null Mutations in a Japanese Population Reproductive Sciences. 2004; 11(2): 118-121

90. Rai P, Kota V, Deendayal M, Shivaji S. Differential proteome profiling of eutopic endometrium from women with endometriosis to understand etiology of endometriosis. J Proteome Res. 2010; 9(9):4407-19.

91. A.G. Braundmeier and A.T. Fazleabas. The non-human primate model of endometriosis: research and implications for fecundityMol. Hum. Reprod 2009;15 (10): 577-586.

92. Armstrong PB, Quigley JP and Sidebottom E. Transepithelial invasion and intramesenchymal infiltration of the chick embryo chorioallantois by tumor cell lines. Cancer Res 1982; 42, 1826-1837.

93. Malik E, Meyhofer-Malik A, Berg C, Bohm W, Kunzi-Rapp K, Diedrich K and Ruck A. Fluorescence diagnosis of endometriosis on the chorioallantoic membrane using 5-aminolaevulinic acid. Hum Reprod 2000; 15,584-588.

94. Maas JW, Groothuis PG, Dunselman GA, de Goeij AF, Struijker-Boudier HA and Evers JL. Development of endometriosis-like lesions after transplantation of human endometrial fragments onto the chick embryo chorioallantoic membrane. Hum Reprod 2001; 16,627-631.

95. Götte, M., Wolf, M., Staebler, A., Buchweitz, O., Kelsch, R., Schüring, A. and Kiesel, L. Increased expression of the adult stem cell marker Musashi-1 in endometriosis and endometrial carcinoma. The Journal of Pathology 2008; 215: 317-329.

96. Christopher L. Coe, Andrine M. Lemieux, Sherry E. Rier, Hideo Uno, and Michele L. Zimbric. Profile of Endometriosis in the Aging Female Rhesus MonkeyJ Gerontol A Biol Sci Med Sci 1998; 53A (1): M3-M7.

97. D'Hooghe TM, Bambra CS, Raeymaekers BM, Koninckx PR. Development of spontaneous endometriosis in baboons. Obstet Gynecol. 1996; 88(3):462-6.

98. Sherry E. Rier, Dan C. Martin, Robert E. Bowman, W. Paul Dmowski and Jeanne L. Becker. Endometriosis in Rhesus Monkeys (Macaca mulatta) Following Chronic

Exposure to 2,3,7,8-Tetrachlorodibenzo-p-dioxin. Toxicol. Sci. 1993; 21 (4): 433-441.

99. Linda C Giudice, Lee C Kao. Endometriosis. Lancet 2004; 364: 1789-99.

100. Fanton JW, Golden JG. Radiation-induced endometriosis in Maccaca mulatta. Radiat Res 1991; 126: 141-46.

101. Rier SE, Martin DC, Bowman RE, et al. Endometriosis in rhesus monkeys (Maccaca mulatta) following chronic exposure to 2,3,7,8 tetrachlorodibenzo-p-dioxin. Fundam Appl Toxicol 1993; 21: 431-41.

102. Koninckx PR, Braet P, Kennedy SH, et al. Dioxin pollution and endometriosis in Belgium. Hum Reprod 1994; 91001-02.

103. Pauwels A, Schepens PJ, D'Hooghe T, Delbeke L, Dhont M, Brouwer A, Weyler J. The risks of endometriosis and exposure to dioxins and polychlorinated biphenyls: a case-controlled study of infertile women. Hum Reprod 2001; 16: 2050-55.

104. Eskenazi B, Mocarelli P, Warner M, et al. Serum dioxin concentrations and endometriosis: a cohort study in Seveso, Italy. Environ Health Perspect 2002; 110: 629-34.

105. Myers JP, Guillette LJ Jr, Palanza P, Parmigiani S, Swan SH, von Saal FS. The emerging science of endocrine disruption. Science and Culture Series. International Seminar on Nuclear War and Planetary Emergencies. 28th Session, 2003, Erice, Italy.

106. Sharpe RM, Franks S. Environment, lifestyle and infertility—an inter-generational issue. Nat Med 2002; suppl 8: s33-40.

107. Welshons WV, Thayer KA, Judy BM, Taylor JA, Curran EM, von Saal FS. Large effects from small exposures, I: mechanisms for endocrine disrupting

chemicals with estrogen activity. Environ Health Perspect 2003; 222: 994–1006

108. Fjerbaek, A. and U.B. Knudsen, Endometriosis, dysmenorrhea and diet--what is the evidence? Eur J Obstet Gynecol Reprod Biol 2007; 132(2): 140-7.

109. Parazzini, F., et al., Selected food intake and risk of endometriosis. Hum Reprod 2004;19(8): 1755-9.

110. Heilier, J.F., et al., Environmental and host-associated risk factors in endometriosis and deep endometriotic nodules: a matched case-control study. Environ Res 2007; 103(1): 121-9.

111. Caserta, D., et al., Impact of endocrine disruptor chemicals in gynaecology. Hum Reprod Update 2008. 14(1): 59-72.

112. Arisawa, K., H. Takeda, and H. Mikasa, Background exposure to PCDDs/PCDFs/PCBs and its potential health effects: a review of epidemiologic studies. J Med Invest 2005; 52(1-2): 10-21.

113. Rier, S.E., et al., Endometriosis in rhesus monkeys (Macaca mulatta) following chronic exposure to 2,3,7,8-tetrachlorodibenzo-p-dioxin. Fundam Appl Toxicol 1993; 21(4): 433-41.

114. Arnold, D.L., et al., Prevalence of endometriosis in rhesus (Macaca mulatta) monkeys ingesting PCB (Aroclor 1254): review and evaluation. Fundam Appl Toxicol 1996; 31(1): 42-55.

115. Yang, J.Z., S.K. Agarwal, and W.G. Foster, Subchronic exposure to 2,3,7,8-tetrachlorodibenzo-p-dioxin modulates the pathophysiology of endometriosis in the cynomolgus monkey. Toxicol Sci, 2000; 56(2): 374-81.

116. Guo, S.W., The link between exposure to dioxin and endometriosis: a critical reappraisal of primate data. Gynecol Obstet Invest 2004; 57(3):157-73.

117. (WHO), W.H.O., Level of PCB's, PCDD's and PCDF's in breast milk: result of WHO coordinated inter-laboratory quality control studies and analytical field studies. WHO Environmental Health Series, 1989.

118. Eskenazi, B., et al., Serum dioxin concentrations and endometriosis: a cohort study in Seveso, Italy. Environ Health Perspect 2002; 110(7): 629-34.

119. Porpora, M.G., et al., Increased levels of polychlorobiphenyls in Italian women with endometriosis. Chemosphere 2006. 63(8): 1361-7.

120. Heilier, J.F., et al., Increased dioxin-like compounds in the serum of women with peritoneal endometriosis and deep endometriotic (adenomyotic) nodules. Fertil Steril 2005; 84(2): 305-12.

121. Cobellis, L., et al., Measurement of bisphenol A and bisphenol B levels in human blood sera from healthy and endometriotic women. Biomed Chromatogr, 2009.

122. Matthew David Rosser. The Emerging Role of Epigenetics in the Aetiology of Endometriosis. MSc thesis/ De Montfort University

123. Degen GH, Bolt HM. Endocrine disruptors: update on xenoestrogens. Int Arch Occup Environ Health. 2000; 73(7):433-41.

124. Morsch DM, Carneiro MM, Lecke SB, Araújo FC, Camargos AF, Reis FM, Spritzer PM. c-fos gene and protein expression in pelvic endometriosis: a local marker of estrogen action. J Mol Histol. 2009;40(1):53-8.

3 BLOOD BIOMARKERS IN ENDOMETRIOSIS

Kannan Kutty and Vidhya Rajkumar

There is an alarming lack of sensitive and specific diagnostic tests for the clinical diagnosis of endometriosis. The clinical presentation varies widely between being severely symptomatic to being completely asymptomatic [1, 2]. This can result in a long delay in the diagnosis of endometriosis that averages from five to eleven years [3]. Additionally, a link between an increase in pain intensity and a decrease in quality of life has been reported in women suffering from endometriosis.

The pressing need for an invasive diagnostic tool, the complex clinical presentation, the diverse morphology of endometriotic lesions, and a shortage of well-designed studies with sufficient number of patients hamper research and delay diagnosis and appropriate treatment for the disease [4].

Discovery of a non-invasive diagnostic test for endometriosis would have a revolutionary impact on the patients' quality of life, the efficiency of existing treatment and the cost of treating the endometriosis. Nevertheless, a recent analysis of 7025 women with endometriosis (European Endometriosis Alliance, 2006) revealed that 65% of them were first undiagnosed or misdiagnosed, and 46% had to seek consultation of many doctors prior to their final correct diagnosis. The diagnosis often involves an average interval of 8 years between the appearance of symptoms and the final diagnosis of the disease [3].

Until now, non-invasive means of diagnosing endometriosis such as ultrasound, magnetic resonance imaging or blood tests have largely failed to produce satisfactory results [5, 6]. But, most of the studies assessing biomarkers for the diagnosis of endometriosis have been beset with several problems: small patient number, frequent need of evaluations of single biomarker, or scant attention of biomarker inconsistencies with regards to the stage of the menstrual cycle [5].

Currently, the diagnosis of endometriosis is only feasible by laparoscopy and biopsy of doubtful lesions with subsequent histological validation of endometriosis; Laparoscopy, although minimally invasive, entails general anesthesia and also surgical expertise in the event of complications. Therefore, it mandates, a non-surgical diagnostic procedure which would be of significant advantage to gynecologists as well as patients. Resolute search to assess the diagnostic value of endometrial biomarkers for endometriosis has been stalled by the dearth of easy, dependable, rapid, accurate and quantitative methods to gauge the levels of these markers in sample material. [7]

Evolving proteomic techniques hold promise of novel strategies to detect biomarkers for the early diagnosis of endometriosis. [7]

It is highly valuable to discover a noninvasive test for early diagnosis which can facilitate instituting early treatment and avert progression. Presently the dismal lack of blood tests for the diagnosis of endometriosis is appalling [5].

In peripheral blood, neither a single biomarker nor a panel of biomarkers has been authenticated as a noninvasive test for endometriosis [8]. It would be obviously advantageous in a clinical setting dealing with women with subfertility with or without pain, a noninvasive test of endometriosis with high sensitivity would be enormously valuable for recognizing those women with endometriosis who could escape from laparoscopic surgery which is credited to provide relief from these symptoms [5, 9]. Desirably, reduced levels of such a biomarker during or post therapy would also associate with lessened pelvic pain and improved fertility. Such a test would expressly be helpful in women with endometriosis, which cannot be detected during gynecological sonography examination.

Blood is an ideal source of biomarkers for reasons more than one. Besides being easily available, it can be used for frequent evaluations and is appropriate for acceptable quantification [5]. The commonly assumed endometriosis bioindicators customarily comprise glycoproteins, growth or adhesion factors, hormones, or with immunology or angiogenesis linked proteins [5].

May et al 2010, conducted using QUADAS (Quality

Assessment of Diagnostic Accuracy Studies) criteria to diagnose endometriosis. This is a methodical review of the literature during the past two and half decades, which evaluates critically the clinical practicality of all projected serum biomarkers for endometriosis in serum, plasma and urine. They identified more than 100 recognized bioindicators in publications that met with the selection criteria. Startlingly they could not pinpoint a single biomarker or panel of biomarkers with undeniable clinical value. While peripheral biomarkers display potential as diagnostic tests, it warrants for more research for acceptance in regular clinical care. It is proposed that panels of markers may help enhance sensitivity and specificity of any diagnostic test. [8]

Serologic testing for CA-125 has been extensively used for discovery of endometriosis and observing advanced disease [10, 11]. Serum levels in women with mild endometriosis are frequently less compared to those in women without endometriosis. A meta-analysis of 23 articles revealed a restricted diagnostic value of serum CA-125 in detecting endometriosis [12].

Plasma levels of CA125 are remarkably high in women with cystic ovarian endometriosis, deeply infiltrating endometriosis or both together;

Although serum CA125 is not a suitable indicator for endometriosis it is useful as a supplementary factor to diagnose endometriosis in patients with chronic pelvic pain. Increased post treatment concentration of CA-125 may serve as a marker of either failure of treatment or relapse of the disease. CA125 assessment in peritoneal fluid entails high sample dilutions or a modified immunoradiometric assay, and hitherto its clinical value has been dubious [12].

Harada T et al 2002 in a retrospective study that

involved 101 women with endometriosis and 22 without it observed that the mean serum CA19-9 concentrations were in patients at all phases of endometriosis . The concentrations were considerably great compared to those without endometriosis. The tinctorial reaction of CA-19-9 was strong in 75% of the samples of endometriotic cysts. This study, endorsed CA19-9 as a suitable indicator for defining the intensity of endometriosis [5].

The suggestion by May et al [8], has been seemingly ratified by Vodolazkaia et al 2012 [13], whose study comprised an aggregate of 28 inflammatory and non-inflammatory plasma bioindicators estimated in 353 plasma samples obtained at surgery. In plasma samples collected during menstruation, multivariate analysis of four biomarkers (annexin V, VEGF, CA-125 and sICAM-1/or glycodelin) aided the diagnosis of US negative endometriosis with a 81–90% sensitivity and a 63–81% specificity in both independent training- and test data set.

The study by SIGNORILE et al 2014 to ascertain specific endometriosis antigens with 2D gel analysis in women with and without endometriosis. Analysis of differentially expressed spots by matrix-assisted laser desorption/ionization-time-of-fl ight/mass spectrometry (nanoLC-ESI-MS/MS) with MASCOT analysis, for detecting the corresponding proteins. ELISAs were performed on a different cohort of endometriosis and healthy patients to validate the differential expression of the identified proteins. Their study ratified the statistical significance of the differential expression of one of these proteins: Zn- alpha2-glycoprotein and recommended analysis of the expression level of this protein in the serum as a novel non-invasive diagnostic test for endometriosis [14].

Paula et al 2015 evaluating the histological variations between eutopic and abdominal wall endometriotic lesions and the expression of mast cell proteases (tryptase and chymase), annexin A1 (ANXA1) and formyl peptide receptor 1 (FPR1).revealed that the endometriotic lesions exhibited a mixed glandular differentiation pattern and a uniform appearance with substantial inflammatory cell infiltration and a noteworthy surge in mast cell proteases -chymase-positive cells and endogenous chymase expression. This clearly correlated with a significant rise and presence of intraepithelial ANXA1 and formyl peptide receptor 1 (FPR1). The joint expression of mast cell chymase and ANXA1-FPR1 system in endometritic lesion implies their participation in the pathogenesis of endometriotic lesions [15].

Proteomics

Innovative advances in molecular biology have led to the use of proteomics in resolving endometriosis. Proteomics helps to comjure thousands of intracelleur proteins, and concomitant findings of any changes in protein expression. These may be of significant clinical germaneness. By virtue of its potential to display the structural and functional profile of proteins, proteomics might shed more light on the nature of the disease. This in turn is much superior to what genomics can reveal. This magnificent modern technology facilitates comparison of not only the expression and regulation profiles of proteins present in endometriosis, but also their comparison with the various phenotypic expressions of endometriosis. Utilization of Proteomic analysis can identify endometriosis-specific proteins, and pathways; in addition. It may serve as a prospective biomarker for precise and early detection. Recent years have witnessed the documentation and comparison of serum and peritoneal fluid protein content in women with and without endometriosis, menstrual blood and urine. It is apparent that proteomics could metamorphose our concept of etiopathogenesis of the disease. Some of the identified proteins could indeed be accountable for the start and evolution of endometriotic implants. As the diagnosis of early phases of endometriosis is difficult. It would be of extreme significance to discover specific biological markers of the disease. Proteomics will add a new dimension to the diagnosis and therapy of endometriosis [16].

Most studies on Proteomics procedures that have been used to diagnose endometriosis, have not been successful thus far. Selection of samples for detection of novel markers (eutopic or ectopic tissue, peritoneal fluid, uterine lavage fluid or blood) combined with the categorization of test samples pose problems. The application of evolving fractionation techniques to capture and concentrate low-abundance proteins, novel -gel-based proteomic technologies vis a vis various protein labeling methods, would catalyse the development of relatively non-invasive diagnostic tests for endometriosis [17].

Li-Hui Zhang 2010, analyzing proteomics of different proteins, observed ectopic and eutopic endometria. One-dimensional electrophoresis together with liquid chromatography and mass spectrometry were used to screen and detect differential proteins .The study embraced five patients with proven endometriosis, five ectopic en-dometria at different stages and five surgically excised eutopic endometria . Three differential bands in one-dimensional electrophoresis were determined by appropriate techniques and 14 up-regulated proteins were discovered. The latter, contained collagen α-1, α-2, α-3(VI), α-1 (XIV) chain, actin, annexin A2, EMILIN-1, ferritin light polypeptide variant, fucosyltransferase 10, myosin-9, protein S100-A9, KIAA1783 protein, and two presumed proteins. They proposed a list of potential biomarkers for endometriosis [18].

Amelie Fassbender et al 2012, verified the validity of the postulate that differential surface-enhanced laser desorption/ionization time-of-flight mass spectrometry protein or peptide found in plasma, can be applied in infertile women to forecast the occurrence of endometriosis, particularly in the subpopulation with a normal preoperative gynecologic ultrasound examination. The study validated that, noninvasive test by proteomic analysis of plasma taken during the menstrual phase, aided the diagnosis of endometriosis undetectable by ultrasonography with great sensitivity and specificity [19].

A plethora of studies have defined signature proteins for the diagnosis of endometriosis [8, 20-22]. A proteomic model, based on three peptide peaks, recorded almost identical sensitivity and specificity to diagnose endometriosis on comparison on 126 cohort of endometriosis patients with 120 healthy controls [21]. In this context it merits mention that PEAKS is a software providing systematic documentation and quantification of entire protein foils. Using raw mass spectrometry findings, PEAKS actively identifies peptide and proteins .PEAKS is equally effective in identifying unrivaled results or confirm ambiguity established by typical database probing [23]. An amalgamation of 5 peptide peaks, exposed by surface-enhanced laser desorption/ionization time-of-flight (SELDI-TOF) mass spectrometry, helped in the diagnosis of endometriosis with highly similar sensitivity and specificity [19]. Despite positive results, these investigations have been encouraging proteomics methods which lack affordability and are relatively slow. [19]. in commencing from raw mass spectrometry instrument data PEAKS effectually in general, the sequence coverage augmented certain of the proteins under investigation.

Actually proteomic technologies warrant further studies for better standardization and reproducibility to be accepted for clinical research projects [24]

Metabolomics

Mainak Dutta et al 2016, making use of mass spectrometry-based lipidomics explored the changes in serum lipid profiles of endometriosis-induced mice. They recognized numerous dysregulated lipids such as phosphatidylcholines, sphingomyelins, phosphatidylethanolamines, and triglycerides. In addition, the study documented that triglycerides possibly are secondary to a general peritoneal inflammatory state. The study also displayed changes in phosphatidylcholine, and found the effect in the ratio of phosphatidylcholine/phosphatidylethanolamine in serum of mice induced with endometriosis. This alteration was possibly attributable to enhanced expression of the phosphatidylethanolamine *N*-methyltransferase gene. The study provides new insight into the etiopathogenesis of endometriosis [25].

Ghazi N et al 2016, conducted a study which focused on the detection of prognostic biomarkers in serum used pattern recognition techniques. The study entailed the use of partial least square discriminant analysis, multi-layer feed forward artificial neural networks (ANNs) and quadratic discriminant analysis (QDA) modeling tools for the early diagnosis of endometriosis in a minimally invasive manner by (1)H- NMR based metabolomics. They collected serum samples from 31 infertile women with laproscopically confirmed endometriosis (stage II and III) and 15 normal women. This was then analyzed by nuclear magnetic resonance spectroscopy. They recorded in endometriotic patients, a remarkable enhancement of the levels of 2- methoxyestron, 2-methoxy estradiol, dehydroepiandrostion androstendione, aldosterone, and deoxy corticosterone. Whereas there was a reduction of cholesterol and primary bile acids levels, there was substantial difference between two study groups. Positive and negative predict value levels were about 71% and 78%, respectively. ANNs also exhibited criteria for diagnosis of endometriosis. Although themodel designed by QDA methods is superior to ANNs in diagnosis of endometriosis, both the methods of modeling have promise of computational aids in noninvasive diagnosis of endometriosis [26].

It is of interest to note that at this juncture the importance and value of urine metabolemic profiling in the non-invasive diagnosis of endometriosis

Sara et al 2015, testedthe significance of urine metabolomic profile to detect biomarkers linked to endometriosis. The investigation comprised 45 endometriosis patients, diagnosed at various phases of the disease, and 36 healthy women. All women had undergone diagnostic laparoscopy to verify the presence of endometriosis. Metabolomic profiling of urine samples based on 1H-nuclear magnetic resonance (NMR) spectroscopy in conjunction with statistical analysis was also conducted. The urine metabolomic profile of endometriosis patients revealed elevated levels of N1- methyl-4-pyridone-5- carboxamide, guanidinosuccinate, creatinine, taurine, valine, and 2-hydroxyisovalerate and reduced levels of lysine compared with healthy women. Most of these metabolites are implicated in inflammation and oxidative stress processes. These pathophysiologic events had been previously described to be present in ectopic endometrial proliferation foci. Generally, the findings suggested that the prospective value of 1H-NMR–based metabolomics, as a quick and noninvasive diagnostic tool to discover metabolic alterations related to endometriosis in urine samples. [27]

Koroshet al 2012, examined the role of omega-3 and omega-6 fatty acids in respect to their potential anti-inflammatory impact on endometriosis. They compared serum phospholipid fatty acid profile in endometriosis patients with controls to test the correlation of this profile with the severity of the disease. The study entailed sixty- four endometriosis patients according to stages of the disease, and seventy four control women, in reproductive age. Various appropriate techniques were employed to determine the fatty acid composition of the phospholipid fraction. Stearic acid in contrast to all other fatty acid components, was strikingly reduced in the endometriosis cohort relative to the controls. It is notable that the serum ratio of eicosapentaenoic acid (EPA) to arachidonic acid (AA) was in sensible proportion with the degree of endometriosis. Overall, the EPA to AA ratio remains a pertinent factor related to showing severity of endometriosis [28].

The usefulness of antiendometrial antibodies and immunoglobulins as biomarkers in the diagnosis of endometriosis is briefly referred to below

Total immunoglobulin

Although endometriosis exerted no impact on the total immunoglobulin levels [29[. El-Roeiy.al not only observed an affirmative association between progressive disease stage and IgG and IgM levels but also a post danazol therapy significant fall in all immunoglobulins studied (IgG, IgM and IgA) [29].

Anti-endometrial antibodies

Endometriosis has been deemed an "autoimmune syndrome". Classical autoimmune diseases, as well as endometriosis, are characterized by polyclonal B-cell activation and production of multiple different autoantibodies [31].

With the advent of identifying antiendometrial antibodies [30].many have reported regular presence of antibodies in women with endometriosis compared to those without endometriosis. Sera from 42 patients with infertility were assessed by indirect immunofluorescence for the presence of antiendometrial antibodies. While 24 out of 28 patients with positive antibody had endometriosis, there was no association between the grade of immunofluorescence and the clinical rigor of endometriosis. Hence, it is considered to have the potential for use as a noninvasive immunological test for endometriosis [32, 33, 34]. The occurrence of anti-endometrial antibodies has been observed in the serum of women with and without endometriosis, however, they have exhibited differential response to disparate antigens in each group [35].

One study reported a sensitivity of 86% and specificity of 76% for the diagnosis of endometriosis in women with infertility or other gynaecological pathology [36].

It has been documented that IgG antibodies exhibited robust association with endometriosis compared to those without endometriosis [30, 37]. A multicentric study of the prospective implication of anti-endometrial antibodies as a bioindicator [38], revealed anti-endometrial antibodies in a big cohort of women who complained of infertility, chronic pelvic pain or dysmenorrhoea: the results were of comparable sensitivity and specificity

Most of the antiendometrial antibodies specially reacted with glands in ectopic and uterine endometrium. Sturdiest antibody reactivity was noted with endometrium from control women, in comparison with uterine and ectopic endometrium from women with endometriosis .It is noteworthy that a fraction of sera with anti-endometrial antibodies also reacted with vascular endothelium and the binding was intense in vaculature in uterine and ectopic endometrium from women with endometriosis relative to endometrium from women without the disease [39].

It has to be appreciated that antiendometrial antibodies per se cannot possibly be a dependable diagnostic parameter of only endometriosis because about 40%–60% of patients with endometriosis have elevated autoantibody titers when tested against a panel of autoantigens [40]. While they often possess specific antiendometrial antibodies [41, 42, 43]. They also exhibit antiovaraian antibodies cAOA, antinuclear autoantibodies (ANA), smooth muscle autoantibodies (SMA), and antiphospholipid antibodies (APA) [44, 45, 46].

References:

[1] Duleba AJ. Diagnosis of endometriosis. Obstetrics and Gynecology Clinics of North America 1997; 24(2):331-346.

[2] Murphy AA. Clinical aspects of endometriosis. Annals of the New York Academy of Sciences 2002; 955:1-10.

[3] Ballard K, Lowton K, Wright J. What's the delay? A qualitative study of women's experiences of reaching a diagnosis of endometriosis. Fertility and Sterility 2006; 86(5):1296-1301.

[4] D'Hooghe T, Debrock S, Mueleman C, Hill JA, Mwenda JA. Future directions in endometriosis research. Obstetrics & Gynecology Clinics of North America.2003; 30:221-244.

[5] Harada T, Kubota T, Aso T. Usefulness of CA19-9 versus CA125 for the diagnosis of endometriosis Fertil Steril. 2002; 78(4): 733-9.

[6] Kennedy S, Bergqvist A, Chapron C, D'Hooghe T, Dunselman G, Greb R, et al. ESHRE guideline for the diagnosis and treatment of endometriosis. Hum Reprod 2005; 20: 2698-704.

[7] Cleophas M Kyama, Sophie Debrock, Jason M Mwenda and Thomas M D'Hooghe. Potential involvement of the immune system in the development of endometriosis. Reproductive Biology and Endocrinology 2003; 1:123.

[8] K. E. May, S. A. Conduit-Hulbert, J. Villar, S. Kirtley, S. H. Kennedy, and C. M. Becker. "Peripheral biomarkers of endometriosis: a systematic review," Human Reproduction Update 2010; 16 (6): 651-674.

[9] D'Hooghe TM, Mihalyi AM, Simsa P, Kyama CK, Peeraer K, De Loecker P, et al. Why we need a noninvasive diagnostic test for minimal to mild endometriosis with a high sensitivity. Gynecol Obstet Invest 2006; 62: 136-8.

[10] Cheng YM, Wang ST and Chou CY. Serum CA-125 in preoperative patients at high risk for endometriosis. Obstet Gynecol 2002; 9: 375-380.

[11] Muyldermans M, Cornillie FJ, Koninckx PR. CA125 and endometriosis. Hum Reprod Update. 1995; 1(2):173-87.

[12] Mol BW, Bayram N, Lijmer JG, Wiegerinck MA, Bongers MY, van der Veen F and Bossuyt PM ,1998 ,The performance of CA-125 measurement in the detection of endometriosis: a meta-analysis. Fertil Steril7 110 1 1108.

[13] A. Vodolazkaia, Y. El-Aalamat, D. Popovic et al. "Evaluation of a panel of 28 biomarkers for the non-invasive diagnosis of endometriosis," Human Reproduction 2012; 27(9): 2698-2711.

[14] Pietro Giulio Signorile and Alfonso Baldi. Blood biomarkers for endometriosis. J. Cell. Physiol 2014; 229: 1731-1735.

[15] Paula R Jr , Oliani AH, Vaz-Oliani DC, D'Ávila SC, Oliani SM, Gil CD. The intricate role of mast cell proteases and the annexin A1-FPR1 system in abdominal wall endometriosis.J Mol Histol. 2015; 46(1):33-43.

[16] Marianowski P, Szymusik I, Hibner M, Barcz E, Wielgoś M. Proteomics in endometriosis]. Ginekol Pol 2013; 84(10):877-81.

[17] Stephens, A. N., Rombauts, L. J. F. and Salamonsen, L. A., 2011. Diagnosis of Endometriosis: Proteomics, in Endometriosis: Science and Practice (eds L. C. Differential Proteomic Analysis of Endometriosis

[18] Li-Hui ZhangHong-Yan LiuHe-Lian Li. Sun MeiChemical Research in Chinese Universities 2010; 26(1).

[19] Amelie Fassbender, Etienne Waelkens, Nico Verbeeck, et al. Level of Evidence: II (Obstet Gynecol 2012; 119:276–85.

[20] X. Long, P. Jiang, L. Zhou, and W. Zhang. "Evaluation of novel serum biomarkers and the proteomic differences of endometriosis and adenomyosis using MALDI-TOF-MS," Archives of Gynecology and Obstetrics 2013; 288 (1): 201–205.

[21] N. Zheng, C. Pan, and W. Liu, 2011,"New serum biomarkers for detection of endometriosis using matrix-assisted laser desorption/ionization time-of-flight mass spectrometry," Journal of International Medical Research, vol. 39, no. 4, pp. 1184–1192, 2011.

[22] A. Fassbender, E. Waelkens, N. Verbeeck, et al,2012,

"Proteomics analysis of plasma for early diagnosis of endometriosis," Obstetrics & Gynecology, vol. 119, no. 2, part 1, pp. 276–285, 2012.

[23] Schmelzer CE1, Schöps R, Ulbrich-Hofmann R, Neubert RH, Raith K.J. Mass spectrometric characterization of peptides derived by peptic cleavage of bovine beta-casein,Chromatogr A. 2004; 5: 1055(1-2):87-92.

[24] A. Fassbender, A. Vodolazkaia, P. Saunders et al. "Biomarkers of endometriosis," Fertility and Sterility 2013; 99(4): 1135–1145.

[25] Mainak Dutta, Mallappa Anitha, Philip B. et al. 2016. Metabolomics Reveals Altered Lipid Metabolism in a Mouse Model of Endometriosis J. Proteome Res., Article ASAPDOI: 10.1021/acs.jproteome.6b00197

[26] Ghazi N, Arjmand M, Akbari Z, Mellati AO, Saheb-Kashaf H, Zamani Z. H NMR-, based metabolomics approaches as non- invasive tools for diagnosis of endometriosis.Int J Reprod Biomed (Yazd). 2016; 14(1):1-8.

[27] Sara Vicente-Mu~noz, Inmaculada Morcillo, Leonor Puchades-Carrasco, et al. 2015, Fertility and Sterility.

[28] Korosh Khanaki, Mohammad Nouri, Ali M. Ardekani, et al. Evaluation of the Relationship between Endometriosis and Omega-3 and Omega-6 Polyunsaturated Fatty Acids Iranian Biomedical Journal 2012; 16 (1): 38-43.

[29] El-Roeiy A, Dmowski W, Gleicher N, Radwanska E, Harlow L, Binor Z, tummon I, Rawlins R. Danazol,1988, but not gonadotropin-releasing hormone agonists suppresses autoantibodies in endometriosis. Fertil Steril. 1988; 50: 864–871.

[30] Mathur S, Garza DE, Smith LF. Endometrial autoantigens eliciting immunoglobulin (Ig)G, IgA, and IgM responses in endometriosis. Fertil Steril. 1990;54:56-63.

[31] Robert Allen Wild, Charles Alex Shivers. Antiendometrial Antibodies in Patients With Endometriosis. American journal of Reproductive Immunology July1985.

[32] Hatayama H, Imai K, Kanzaki H, Higuchi T, Fujimoto M, Mori T. Detection of antiendometrial antibodies in patients with endometriosis by cell ELISA. Am J Reprod Immunol. 1996; 35:118-122.

[33] Meek S, Hodge D, Musich J. Autoimmunity in infertile patients with endometriosis. Am J Obstet Gynecol. 1988; 158: 1365-1373.

[34] Bohler HC, Gercel-Taylor C, Lessey BA, Taylor DD. Endometriosis markers: immunologic alterations as diagnostic indicators for endometriosis. Reprod Sci. 2007; 14: 595-604.

[35] Rajkumar K, Malliah V, Simpson CW. Identifying the presence of antibodies against endometrial antigens: a preliminary study. J Reprod Med. 1992; 37:552-556.

[36] Wild RA, Shivers CA. Antiendometrial antibodies in patients with endometriosis. Am J Reprod Immunol Microbiol. 1985; 8:84-86.

[37] Odukoya OA, Wheatcroft N, Weetman AP, Cooke ID. The prevalence of endometrial immunoglobulin G antibodies in patients with endometriosis. Hum Reprod. 1995a; 10: 1214-1219.

[38] Randall GW, Gantt PA, Poe-Zeigler RL, Bergmann CA, Noel ME, Strawbridge WR, Richardson-Cox B,

Hereford JR, Reiff RH. Serum antiendometrial antibodies and diagnosis of endometriosis. Am J Reprod Immunol 2007; 58:374-382.

[39] Fernández-Shaw S[1], Hicks BR, Yudkin PL, Kennedy S, Barlow DH, Starkey PM. Anti-endometrial and anti-endothelial auto-antibodies in women with endometriosis. Hum Reprod. 1993; 8(2):310-5.

[40] S. Vassiliadis, K. Relakis, A. Papageorgiou, and I. Athanassakis. "Endometriosis and infertility: a multi-cytokine imbalance versus ovulation, fertilization and early embryo development," Clinical & Developmental Immunology 2005; 12(2): 125-129.

[41] L. Harborne, R. Fleming, H. Lyall, J. Norman, and N. Sattar. "Descriptive review of the evidence for the use of metformin in polycystic ovary syndrome," Lancet 2003; 361(9372): 1894–1901.

[42] D. I. Lebovic, M. D. Mueller, and R. N. Taylor. "Immunobiology of endometriosis," Fertility and Sterility 2001; 75(1): 1–10.

[43] M. B. Goldman and D. W. Cramer. "The epidemiology of endometriosis," Progress in Clinical and Biological Research 1990; 323: 15–31.

[44] E. Geva, A. Amit, L. Lerner-Geva, and J. B. Lessing. "Autoimmunity and reproduction," Fertility and Sterility 1997; 67(4): 599–611.

[45] R. L. Kelkar, P. K. Meherji, S. S. Kadam, S. K. Gupta, and T. D. Nandedkar. "Circulating auto-antibodies against the zona pellucida and thyroid microsomal antigen in women with premature ovarian failure," Journal of Reproductive Immunology 2005; 66(1): 53–67.

[46] J. M. Wheeler. "Epidemiology of endometriosis-

associated infertility," The Journal of Reproductive Medicine 1989; 34 (1): 41–46.

4 IMAGING ENDOMETRIOSIS

Associate Professor Dr Marymol Koshy;
Radiologist,
Faculty of Medicine, Universiti Teknologi MARA, Malaysia

Introduction

Noninvasive imaging modalities can assist in the diagnosis of endometriosis but ultimately the diagnosis is confirmed or refuted on laparoscopy along with histological evaluation of the excised lesion(s). In this chapter we will discuss the various imaging modalities used for the evaluation of endometriosis, the strengths and weaknesses of the various modalities and their method or protocol.

The workup of endometriosis actually begins with a detailed history and physical examination. When it comes to imaging endometriosis, pelvic ultrasound scanning is the initial imaging examination, mainly because it is a non-invasive test that is inexpensive and readily available in most centers. However Magnetic resonance imaging (MRI) provides far superior anatomic details and better definition of abnormalities than ultrasound although it is costly and easily accessible.

Radiologists often use the terms endometriosis and endometriomas interchangeably. However, it is important to remember that endometriomas constitute only a part of the disease process known as endometriosis, which also includes endometriotic implants (peritoneal and extraperitoneal) and adhesions [1].

There are three forms of pelvic endometriosis. The first form is the superficial endometriosis or Sampson syndrome. Superficial peritoneal lesion(s) or non-invasive implants are best seen on laparoscopy, as these lesions are usually too small to detect on non-invasive imaging. Second is the endometriomas, which is the localized form of endometriosis and is also known as chocolate cyst or endometriotic cyst. The cysts are usually 2-5 cm in size, however they may be up to 20 cm in size. Due to repeated cyclical hemorrhage it contains dark degenerated blood products. Endometriomas are most commonly located in the ovaries, however they can also be found in other sites such as the anterior/posterior cul-de-sac, posterior broad ligament, uterosacral ligament, uterus and colon (Table 1). The main role of the radiologists is to detect and evaluate endometriomas as the radiological evaluation of small endometriotic implants is limited.

COMMON SITES OF ENDOMETRIOMAS	
1	Ovaries
2	Anterior cul-de-sac
3	Posterior cul-de-sac
4	Posterior broad ligament
5	Uterosacral ligament
6	Uterus
7	Colon

Table 1. Common sites of endometriomas

The third form is deep or solid infiltrating pelvic endometriosis. Deeply infiltrating endometriosis (DIE) is considered as a specific entity, which has been arbitrarily defined in histological terms as endometriotic lesions extending more than 5 mm underneath the peritoneum [2]. It can affect fibromuscular pelvic structures, such as the rectovaginal septum and uterosacral ligaments (69.2% of cases), as well as the vagina (14.5%), alimentary tract (9.9%), urinary tract (6.4%), and other extraperitoneal pelvic sites [3]. Patients with deep pelvic endometriosis have more severe symptoms and the symptoms, needless to reiterate, are usually related to the localization and depth of invasion.

Intestinal evaluation of deep endometriotic lesions is extremely important as the number and depth of lesions influence the surgical planning and approach. Bowel involvement is frequently multifocal, and the most commonly affected areas are the rectosigmoid colon, the appendix, the caecum, and the distal ileum [4].
Bladder and ureteral involvement also influence surgical management of endometriosis. Bladder involvement is usually described as extrinsic or intrinsic involvement. In extrinsic involvement the endometriotic implants are generally confined to the serosal surface. In intrinsic involvement there is infiltration of the muscular layers, which are seen as mural masses projecting into the lumen. These masses are most of the time near the dome of the bladder and can be indistinguishable from a neoplasm in which case cystoscopy with biopsy is required for definitive diagnosis.

Endometriosis has been reported in unusual sites such as the chest and abdominal wall. Abdominal wall endometriosis usually occurs near a cesarean section scar.

Plain radiography

As the symptoms of endometriosis are variable, a diverse array of imaging studies may be done including plain radiography, barium studies and intravenous urography. The findings from plain radiography or contrast studies such as barium enema or intravenous urography are nonspecific. The circumstances under which these imaging studies are done are as follows.

Plain radiography has no role in the radiologic workup of endometriosis, as there are no specific findings.
Chest endometriosis may present as pneumothorax, haemothorax and lung nodules on plain radiograph.

Women with rectal pain or bleeding due to endometriosis involvement of the bowel may undergo barium enema contrast study. The appearance of gastrointestinal implants on double-contrast barium enema images is variable, but the involvement is often asymmetric, with puckering or a crenulated appearance of the affected wall [5]. A typical finding is that of a tethered submucosal mass at the center of the anterior midrectum, which represents cul-de-sac implants involving the rectal wall. Rectal carcinoma or serosal metastases can mimic the appearance of endometriosis on barium enema. In deep infiltrating endometriosis of the bowel wall, patients may present with constipation or pencil-like stool as a result of circular endometriotic involvement. This may be seen as an area of stenosis of the bowel lumen on barium enema contrast study.

An intravenous urography examination in patients with endometriosis may show ureteral obstruction at or below the pelvic brim. This obstruction may either be from an invasion of an endometriosis implant into the ureter or due to the mass effect of an endometrioma.

The findings from plain radiography or contrast studies such as barium enema or intravenous urography are nonspecific.

Ultrasound

Patients referred for ultrasound, when endometriosis is suspected must have both a transvesicular and transvaginal study. A transvaginal study is more sensitive for detecting small endometriomas, bladder lesions and deep nodules such as those in the rectovaginal septum. The kidneys must be also be scanned to exclude hydroureter and hydronephrois. The experience of the operator can also exert profound influence on the results.

Ultrasound is predominantly used to evaluate the ovaries. When an ovarian cyst is detected it should be completely characterized and evaluated by determining its wall morphology, internal echogenicity and its effect on the surrounding structures. As the cul-de-sac is commonly involved, care must be taken to completely scan this area.

There is a wide spectrum in the sonographic appearances of endometriomas. Endometriomas may be uni or multilocular and may contain thin or thick septations. A multilocular endometrioma may consist of multiple separate cysts with thin or thick septations between these loculi. They may appear as simple or complex cystic masses or they may even resemble a solid mass (Fig 1). The presence of old blood gives a ground glass appearance with low-level echoes. A characteristic finding of endometrioma is a cystic mass with diffuse low-level echoes (Fig 2). Very rarely they can appear as anechoic cysts, mimicking a functional ovarian cyst.

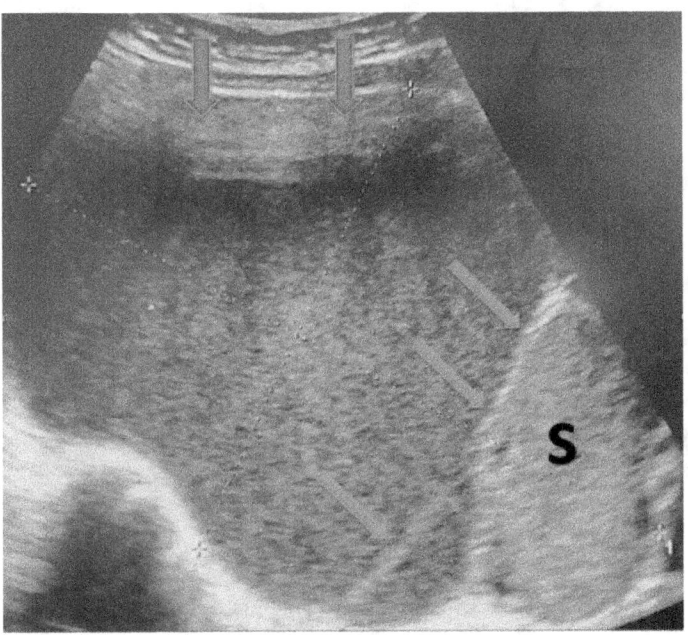

Fig 1. Transabomimnal ultrasound of a multilocular endometrioma consisting of separate cysts with septations (blue arrow). The larger cysts shows a heterogeneous appearance, with diffuse, low-level echoes interspersed with echogenic and anechoic areas. Note the diffuse wall thickening (red arrows), which can be a feature of endometrioma. The smaller cyst resembles a solid mass (S).

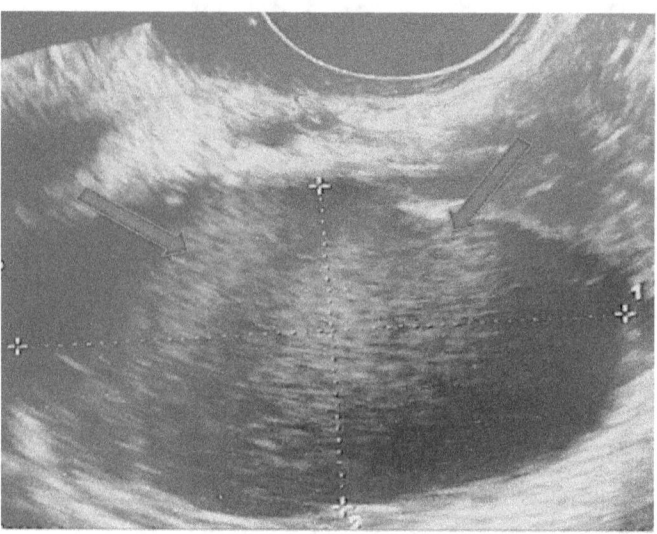

Fig 2. Transvaginal ultrasound of an endometrioma (arrows) showing the characteristic diffuse low-level echoes

Attention must be focused on o the endometrial cyst wall as it can have variable presentations. Features such diffuse wall thickening, wall nodularity and echogenic foci within the cyst may be present. Patel et al found no diagnostic value in the assessment of wall thickness for differentiating between endometriomas and other ovarian masses. In their study, 20% of endometriomas had solid-appearing wall nodularity, a feature that is classically associated with neoplasia [6].

Although not commonly seen punctate echogenicities or echogenic foci, if present in the wall of the endometriorias increases the specificity of the diagnosis. However if not carefully searched for, these deposits can be easily missed. Echogenic foci seen adherent to the wall have been postulated to be cholesterol deposits (Fig 3) however, they may also be small blood clots or debris (Fig 4). When detected these foci must be differentiated from wall nodules. It is important to highlight that these nodules may be precancerous and hence the need to distinguish the difference.

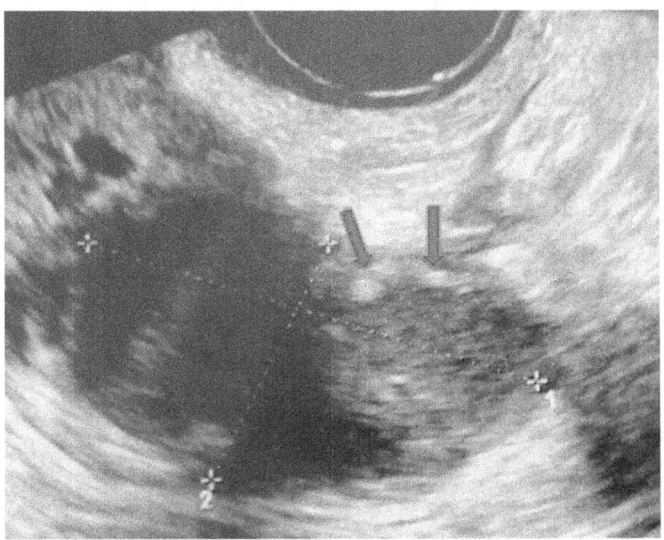

Fig 3. Transvaginal ultrasound: Multilocular ovarian endometrioma with echogenic wall foci consistent with cholesterol deposits (red arrows)

As ultrasound scan characteristics of endometriomas overlap with other pathologies. Differential diagnosis of endometriomas includes dermoid cysts, hemorrhagic cysts, ovarian abscesses and cystic neoplasms. With careful analysis ultrasound can help narrow the differential diagnosis. Dermoid cysts when compared with endometiomas have distinct features such as calcification, fat-fluid levels, and hyperechoic areas. In the case of acute haemorrhagic cyst, patient history may be useful as haemorrhagic cysts are usually acute in presentation as opposed to endometriosis. Haemorrhagic cysts usually appear as complex cysts, with clot retraction and fibrin stranding. The fibrin strands may mimic septations but these strands are usually thinner and weaker reflectors when compared with true septations. Haemorrhagic cysts mostly resolve within 4-6 weeks, so if the mass resolves on follow-up examination, endometrioma can be safely ruled out. Cystic neoplasm may resemble septate endometrioma however on ultrasound Doppler, color flow will be seen in septations. When compared with benign lesions, endometriomas are often multiple or bilateral increasing their resemblance to malignancies. If the cyst has a solid or soft tissue component, malignancy must be excluded. Ultrasound Doppler waveform analysis is of little value in detecting endometriomas as Low-resistance waveforms encountered in endometriomas are also seen in malignancy.

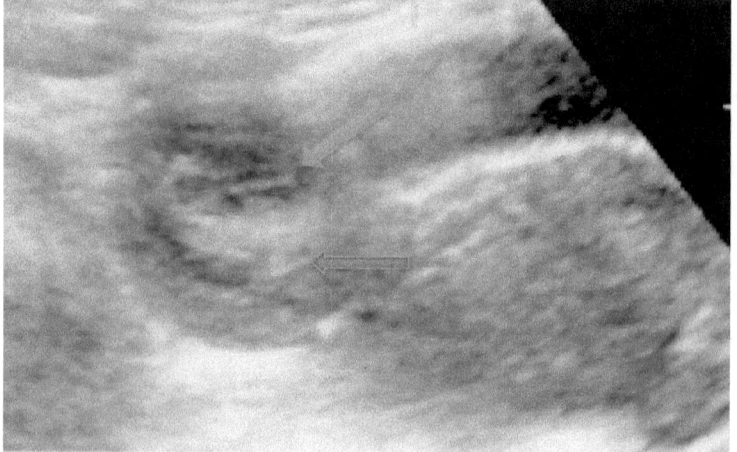

Fig 4. Transabdominal ultrasound showing a cystic lesion with hyperechoic structure within. This turned out to be an ovarian endometrioma with clot and debris (Red arrow).

In using transvaginal ultrasound for detecting deep endometriotic lesions, the examiner must be able to visualize the bladder wall, the pouch of Douglas, the vaginal wall and the rectovaginal septum, the rectosigmoid, the retrocervical (uterosacral ligaments and torus uterinus), and paracervical areas (ureteral involvement). Deep endometriotic lesions may be seen as round hypoechoeic areas infiltrating the organ wall or region. Some of these lesions may contain hyperechoic foci. On pressing the transducer against the lesion, the patient may experience deep pain. The accuracy in the detection of deep endometriotic lesions on transvaginal ultrasound depends on the location of the lesion.

Studies have evaluated the need of specific preparation for transvaginal scanning, such as rectal aqueous contrast, bowel preparations with laxatives, and vaginal injection of gel. It is not conclusive whether these techniques enhance the performance of the test or should be routinely used [7]. Hudelist et al. analyzed the diagnostic value of transvaginal sonography for noninvasive, presurgical detection of bowel endometriosis and concluded that transvaginal ultrasound with or without the use of prior bowel preparation is an accurate test for noninvasive, presurgical detection of deep infiltrating endometriosis of the rectosigmoid [8]. If paracervical lesions are detected on transvaginal ultrasound, ureteral involvement has to be excluded. Ureteral obstruction by endometriosis can lead to hydroureter and/or hydronephrosis, which can eventually lead to renal failure. Hence a urinary tract ultrasound followed by renal function tests may be judicious.

Ultrasound is not sensitive in detecting small peritoneal implants. Although ultrasound is unable to detect adhesions it is able to assess mobility and fixation.

In patients with suspected bowel endometriosis transvaginal ultrasound is the first choice of imaging investigation. Although transrectal ultrasound has not shown to be superior to transvaginal ulatrasound, it can be used to detect posterior bladder wall lesions and also to demonstrate rectal involvement.

In abdominal wall endometriosis ultrasound shows solid hypoechoeic lesions in the abdominal wall. On ultrasound Doppler examinations, these lesions may contain internal vascularity. However the ultrasound findings are non-specific and a diverse spectrum of diseases has to be considered in the differential diagnosis including hernia, haematoma, abscess, suture granuloma and malignancies such as sarcoma, desmoids tumour or metastasis.

Recently, the use of three-dimensional transvaginal ultrasound (3D TVUS) for the diagnosis of DIE was reported, with good results for vaginal lesions. However, analysis of sensitivity and specificity of 3D TVUS for the diagnosis of DIE in specific sites suggests no striking improvement in comparison to two-dimensional transvaginal ultrasound [9. 10]. In summary the classical finding of endometriosis is a cystic mass with diffuse low-level echoes. The wall may also have nodules, which is also a feature of ovarian neoplasms. Nevertheless ,, if the mural nodules are hyperechoic they then have a high predictive value for endometrioma over non-endometrial lesions [11]. Other appearances are much less specific and can be mimicked by hemorrhagic cysts, tubo-ovarian abscesses, and cystadenomas. Due to the wide variability of appearances on ultrasound, endometriomas are considered to be the most difficult adnexal lesion to diagnose.

Patient preparation and procedure

Transvaginal ultrasound examination should be performed using an ultrasound machine with 5–9-MHz frequency transducer. Ideally it should be performed following bowel preparation. Bowel preparation is done to eliminate faecal content and gas in the rectosigmoid colon.

Bowel preparation, if contemplated, consists of a low-residue diet 24 hours before the examination and a laxative that can be administered in oral doses before the scheduled transvaginal ultrasound examination.

Alternatively an enema can be administered approximately 1 hour before the examination.

The scan must include the evaluation of the uterus, ovaries, bladder wall, anterior uterine seorsa, uterine insertion of the round ligaments, rectovaginal septum and posterior vaginal fornix. The pelvic peritoneum covering the bladder, uterus, Douglas pouch, retrocervical region and rectosigmoid colon must also be evaluated. Rectosigmoid colon evaluation must be done from the anal verge to the sigmoid-descending colon transition. This can be done by moving the transducer up and down and turning the transducer in the axial and sagittal planes.

As the descending colon, appendix, and ileocecal transition are inaccessible transvaginally, these structures must be assessed by transabdominal ultrasound using a linear-array transducer. This should be performed following the transvaginal ultrasound. Due to the presence of gas and fecal residues in the ileocecal segment, detecting endometriotic lesions in the descending colon may impair the accuracy of the ultrasound findings

Ultrasound examination of the intestinal lesion must determine which layer of the wall is affected. On ultrasound normal intestinal wall depicted from outer to inner layer consist of a thin hyperechoic line representing the serosa; two hypoechoic strips separated by a thin hyperechoic line representing the muscularis propria; a hyperechoic line representing submucosa; a hypoechoic line representing muscularis mucosa and a hyperechoic linear interface between the bowel lumen and mucosa.

Computed tomography (CT) scan

The appearance of endometriosis is non-specific on computed tomography (CT) scans and hence, it is not performed typically in the radiologic evaluation of endometriosis.

On CT scan endometriomas may appear as cystic masses (Fig 5). The finding on CT scan of a hyperdense focus inside an ovarian cyst is suggestive of endometrioma and should help distinguish endometrioma from other pelvic masses [12].

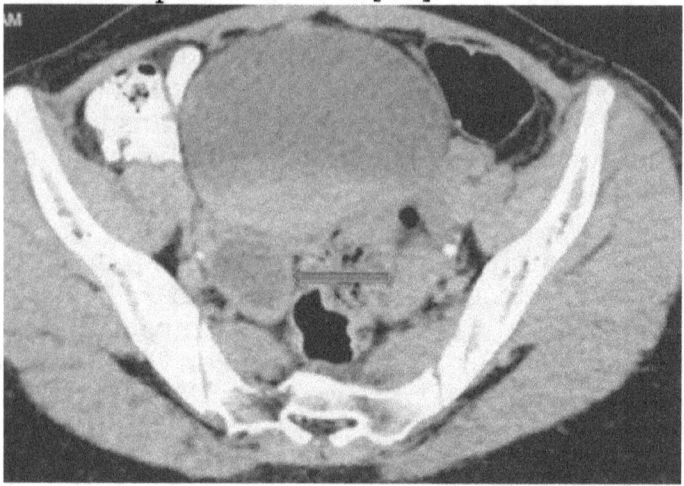

Fig 5. CT Scan showing a predominantly cystic mass in the right adnexal region representing an ovarian endometrioma

Complications of endometriosis caused by adhesions in the form of bowel obstruction or ureteral obstruction causing hydronephrois may be evident on CT scans. Endometriotic implants involving the urinary bladder that infiltrate the muscle and appear as mural masses projecting into the lumen of the bladder can be detected by CT scans.

CT scan findings in abdominal wall endometriosis are nonspecific. They can present as cystic or solid enhancing masses within the abdominal wall. An inflammatory reaction may be seen as tissue stranding surrounding the border of the mass on CT (Fig 6).

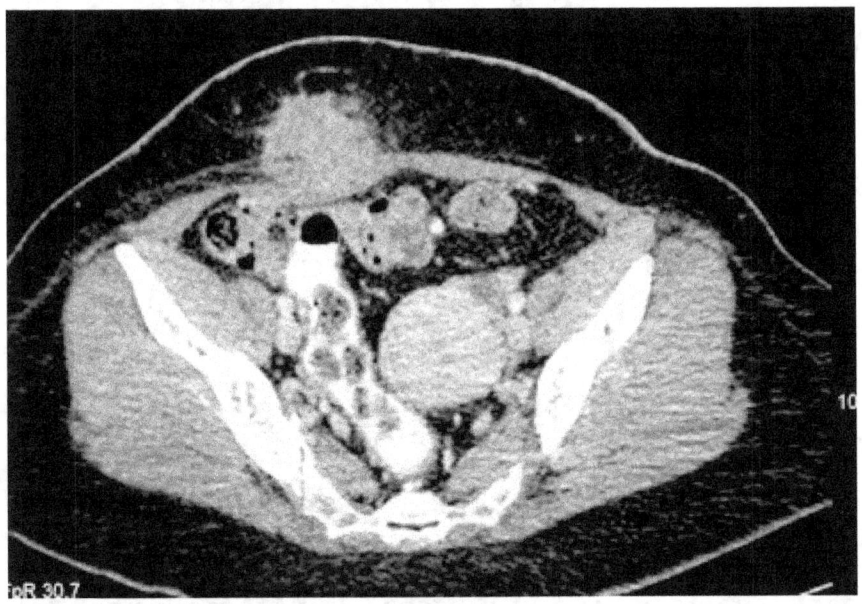

Fig 6. Rectus muscle enodmetrioma in a 42 year old with history of lump in her anterior abdominal wall. Axial CT scan shows a solid mass with surrounding tissue stranding.

Pelvic inflammatory disease or ovarian tumours can easily mimic the appearance of endometriomas or enodmetriosis on CT scan. Hence CT scan cannot be relied on for the diagnosis of endometriosis.

Magnetic resonance imaging (MRI)

Although laparoscopic biopsy with histological confirmation is the gold standard for diagnosing endometriosis, MRI is increasingly being used, especially to evaluate deep disease, with high sensitivity o of 90

% and specificity of 91% [13]. Extension of deep infiltrating enodmetriosis can be determined especially when adhesions are present, as adhesions can limit laparoscopic inspection.

Superficial endometriosis are non-invasive implants which are scattered across the peritoneum, ovaries and uterine ligaments. On laparoscopy, based on the degree of haemorrhage, scarring and fibrosis within the implants they can be white, black or red. As these lesions are small and flat they are usually not detected by MRI. Small nonhemorrhagic lesions can easily escape detection with MRI. Lesions more than 5mm and haemorrhagic cysts which show hyperintensity on T1-weighted (T1W) images and hypointensity on T2-weighted (T2W) images can be detected with MRI. Larger fibrotic implants can be seen as speculated nodules of very low signal intensity on T2W images. The commonest site for implants is the cul-de-sac, however they can also be seen on the dome of the bladder, rectum, umbilicus or pelvic surgical scars. On T1W fat saturated images, haemorrhage, if present within these lesions can be seen as punctuate high signal intensities. As MRI is not sensitive for superficial implants it should not be relied on to rule out endometriosis.

On MRI, endometriomas can present as solitary or multilocular masses (Fig 7) with diverse appearances as it depends on the concentration of iron and protein in the fluid, and also the products of blood degradation.

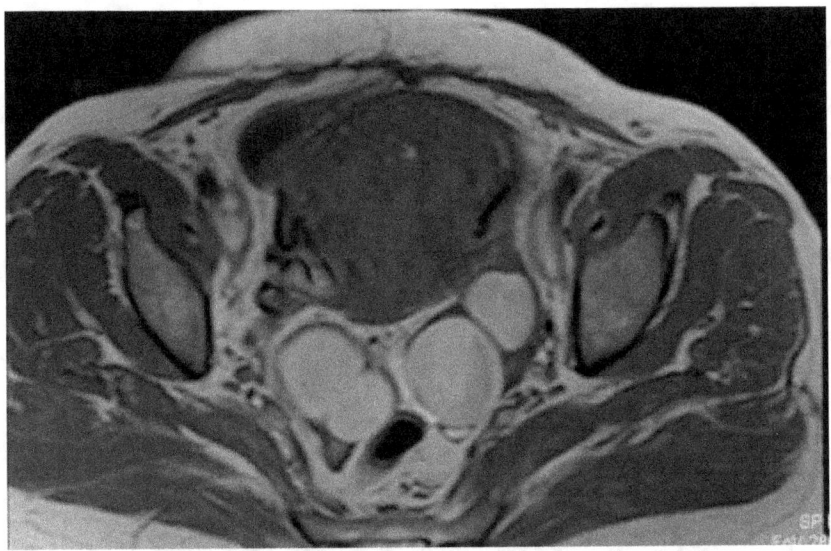

Fig 7. Bilateral multilocular endometrioma on T1-weighted image.

The gross appearance of most endometriomas is chocolate cysts due to the high concentration of blood products. On MRI these endometriomas will be demonstrated as cystic masses with homogeneous hyperintense signal intensity on T1W (Fig 8) and T1W fat saturation sequences. The T1W fat saturation helps differentiate endometriomas from mature cystic teratomas, which usually contain fat (Fig 9).
On T2W images, endometriomas may range from having a low signal intensity, which is termed as shading, to intermediate, or high signal intensity (Fig 10). The low signal intensity reflects the hemoconcentration in the enodmetrioma and is a feature rarely seen in other masses (Fig 11). Endometriomas generally have a thick, fibrous capsule with low signal intensity on T2W, caused by hemosiderin-laden macrophages (Fig 12).

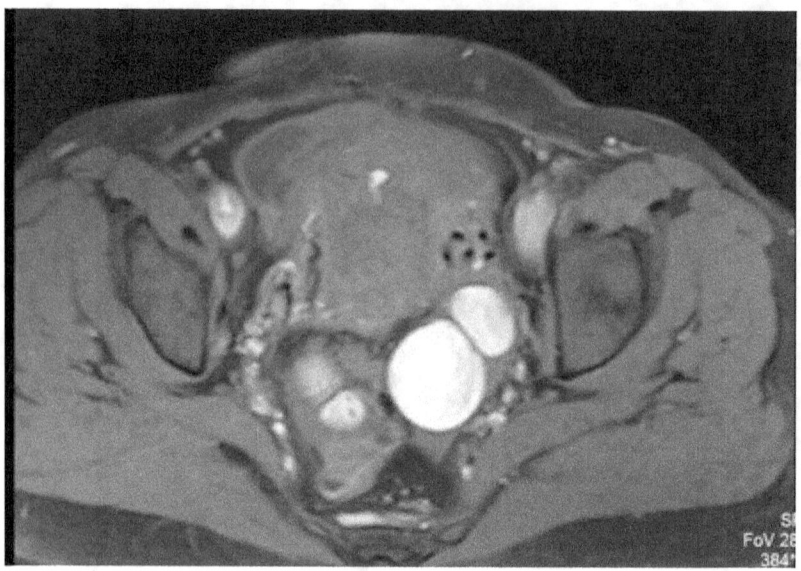

Fig 8. T1W fat saturation image of an endometrioma with hyperintense blood

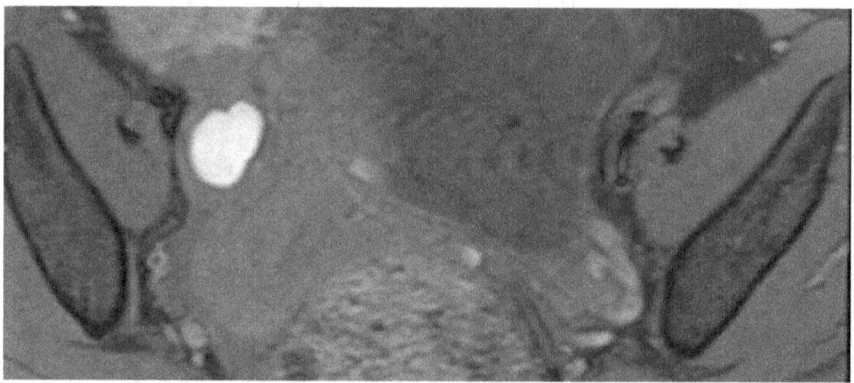

Fig 9. Axial T1-weighted fat-suppressed image reveals right ovarian endometrioma that appears hyperintense. Mature cystic teratoma will also show high signal on T1-weighted images however on fat suppressed there is loss of signal differentiating it from endometriomas, which remain high.

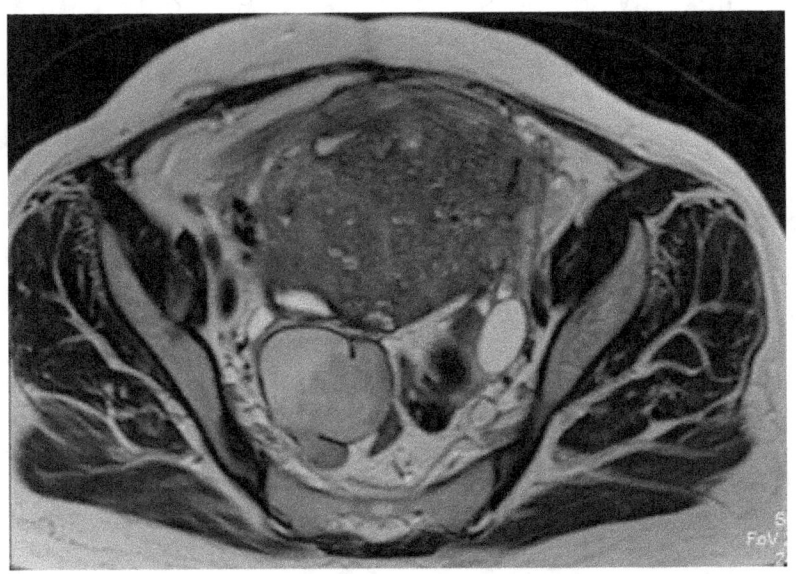

Fig 10. On T2W image, endometriomas may range from having a low signal intensity (arrow) which is also known as shading, to an intermediate or high signal intensity. Shading depends on the concentration of the blood products. Also note diffuse uterine adenomyosis.

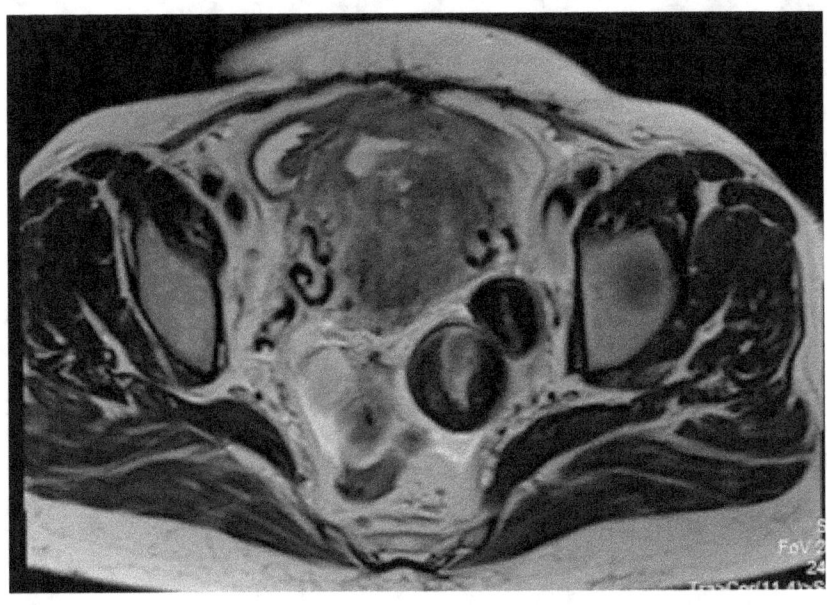

Fig 11. The T2W image shows an endometrioma with a bloodclot, which is hypointense on T2. These clots can be accompanied by fibrotic tissue at histopathology.

On T1W images, ovaries showing multiple high signal lesions are highly suggestive of endometriosis. Aside from endometrioma an adnexal mass with high signal intensity on T1W images include haemorrhagic functional ovarian cyst and mature cystic teratoma. In 1993, Outwater et al compared the MR imaging features of endometriomas and hemorrhagic cysts and concluded that endometriomas tended to have higher T1W and lower T2W signal intensities than hemorrhagic cysts [14]. The greater degree of T1 and T2 shortening in endometriomas is attributable to their higher protein concentration and viscosity.

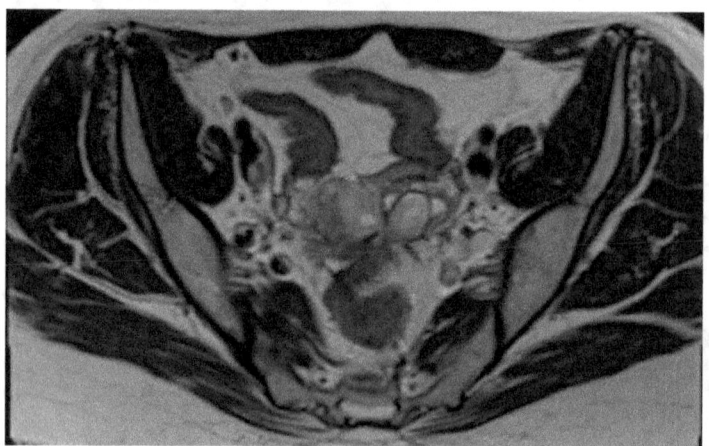

Fig 12. Axial T2- weighted image shows an endometrial cyst of the left ovary. The wall of the cyst shows a peripheral rim of low signal intensity on T2WI representing hemosiderin or fibrous capsule.

MRI is useful for both the diagnosis of deep infiltrating endometriotic lesions and to determine the extension of the disease. Preoperative assessment of disease extension is essential especially when deciding if surgical intervention is indicated, and if so, in planning of surgical excision.

Histology of the disease entity of deep endometriosis is required to better understand the signal intensity characteristics at MR imaging. The main characteristic of deep endometriosis on microscopic examination is fibromuscular hyperplasia surrounding sparse ectopic endometrial glands. The endometrial glands and stroma infiltrate the adjacent fibromuscular tissue and elicit smooth muscle proliferation and fibrous reaction, resulting in the formation of solid nodules [15, 16]. The ectopic endometrial foci, as well as eutopic endometrium, respond to hormonal stimulation with various degrees of cyclic hemorrhage. The episodes of bleeding within these foci result in a variable inflammatory response and fibrous reaction [17]. Relatively acellular regions of fibrous tissue, as well as compact smooth muscle, have intermediate signal intensity on T1W MR images and low signal intensity on T2W images [18]. Consequently, on T2W images, solid endometriotic masses or nodules will appear as hypointense masses with irregular, indistinct, or stellate margins due to the presence of abundant fibrous tissue and smooth muscle proliferation. Deep endometriotic lesions may also be depicted as irregular and predominantly hypointense soft-tissue thickening with T2W sequences [17].

In visceral solid endometriosis, these implants adhere to the serosal surface of the bowel and may invade the muscular layers, eliciting marked smooth muscle proliferation. Stricture formation and obstruction may result [3].

The cul-de-sac is the most common site of deep infiltrating endometriosis and it can be easily overlooked at laparoscopy. MRI can readily differentiate normal anatomy and presence of endometriosis in the cul-de-sac. The posterior fornix and the torus uterinus where the sacrouterine ligaments attach are common sites of endometriosis. These patients usually present with dyspareunia.

MRI is useful in bowel endometriosis as it can determine the depth of bowel wall infiltration, the distance of the affected area from the anus and its length.

Deep infiltrating endometriosis should be suspected when the sacrouterine ligaments or rectal wall have hypointense thickened or nodular appearances on T2W images

Endometriosis can be complicated by adhesions. Adhesions can cause fixation of the pelvic organs, which can lead to posterior displacement of the uterus and ovaries, elevation of the posterior vaginal fornix and angulation of bowel loops. Complications such as hydronephrosis can be caused by adhesions. As a result of extensive adhesion formation ovaries can get stuck together known as 'kissing ovaries' (Fig 13).

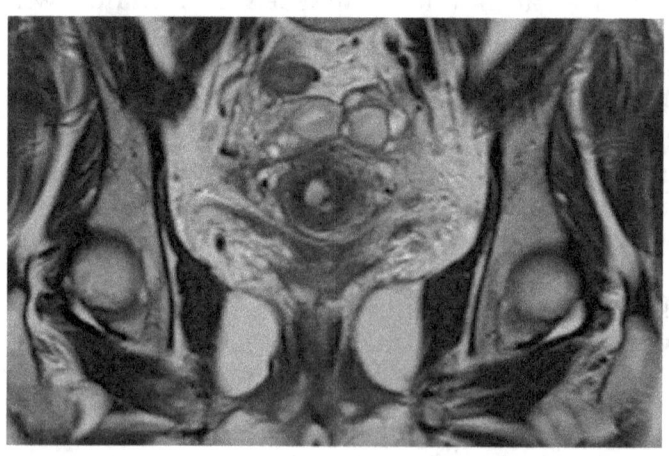

Fig 13. Coronal T2W images showing kissing ovaries due to adhesions

As in CT scan, MRI findings in abdominal wall endometriosis are nonspecific, showing a solid enhancing mass within the abdominal wall. On T1W fat saturation image these masses have a slightly higher signal intensity to muscle. On T2W image the masses have an isointense signal to muscle. Small foci of high signal intensities may be seen within the mass representing dilated endometrial glands (Fig 14).

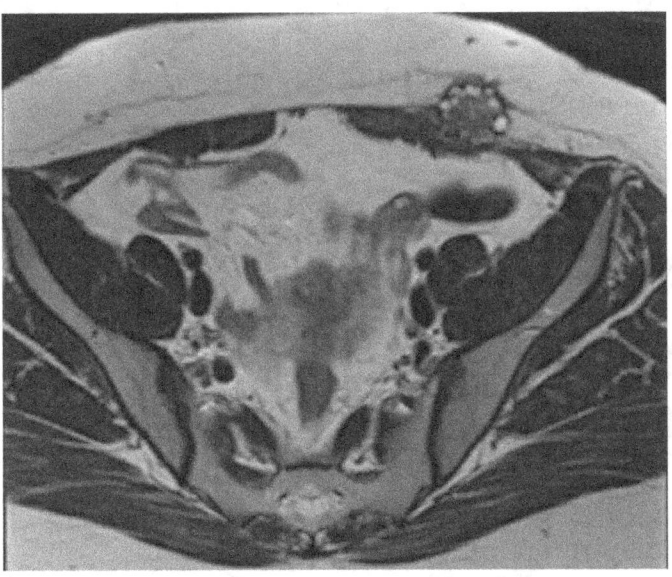

Fig 14. Abdominal wall endometriosis: On T2WI, the lesions have an isointense signal to muscle with small foci of high signal intensity, indicating dilated endometrial glands.

In patients with endometriosis dilated fallopian tubes can be seen as high signal intensities on T1W images indicating bloody fluid. Debris may be seen at the dependent portions of the tube. Sometimes a complicated hydrosalpinx may be the only imaging finding indicating endometriosis [19].

Complications of endometriosis such as bowel implants and ureteral obstruction can be demonstrated on MRI.

MRI Protocol

MR imaging can be performed at any stage of the patient's menstrual cycle. However, the date of the patient's last menstrual period should be recorded for interpretation purposes.

Antiperistaltic medications (unless contraindicated) such as 1 mg of glucagon intramuscularly or scopolamine-*N*-butyl bromide intravenously can be administered to reduce motion artifacts due to bowel peristalsis. Fasting for at least 6 hours prior to MRI can help visualize the bowel better especially since long imaging time is required for MRI. 50 mL of intravaginal aqueous gel can be administered. This will distend the vaginal cavity and allow better assessment of both the vaginal fornices and the retrocervical region. In patients where rectal involvement is suspected endorectal gel or saline solution can be administered.

The bladder should neither be underfilled nor distended. A distended bladder can cause phase ghost artifacts and compress the uterus. Ghosting from respiratory motion artifact can be dimished by placing saturation bands along the anterior and posterior body wall fat.

MRI must be performed using a dedicated pelvic coil as these external multicoil arrays provide a high signal-to-noise ration resulting in improved spatial resolution. Aside from that it also enhances anatomic details. The imaging planes must include all three standard projections, which are axial, sagittal and coronal. The sagittal plane is most helpful in evaluating the cul-de-sac and rectum.

In addition to T1W and T2W pulse sequences it is recommended that all MR imaging of the female pelvis include a T1W fat suppressed sequence for two reasons. Firstly on T1W images endometriomas have relatively homogenous high signal intensity similar to or greater than that of fat. As fat saturation narrows the dynamic signal range, differences in tissue signal will be accentuated. Removal of high signal intensity of surrounding fat will enable more sensitive detection of smaller endometriomas. Secondly T1W images with fat suppression can differentiate blood in endometriomas from fat in mature cystic teratomas as both show high signal intensity on T1W images without fat suppression.

If MRI is performed to determine the presence or extent of endometriosis then T1W images with fat suppression in axial and sagittal planes with T2W images in axial, sagittal and coronal planes will suffice. Post gadolinium images have not been found to be particularly useful in the detection of endometriomas. There is no role of gadolinium in the detection of small implants as enhancing small vessels can be mistaken as endometriotic deposits. However in the case of more diverse disease or suspected malignancy, T1W and T1W fat saturation sequences before and after the administration of intravenous gadolinium must be added. Post gadolinium images are best acquired beginning 10 seconds after the injection as the lesion(s) yields the most information. Diffusion-weighted imaging may also be supplemented.

Generally endometriosis will be demonstrated as low to intermediate signal intensities on T1W and T2W images. Dilated endometrial glands may be seen as punctuate foci of high signal intensity on T2W images. T1W images with fat saturation are the most sensitive for the detection of haemorrhage, which can be seen as high signal intensity areas. High-resolution T2W sequences are used for the evaluation of fibrotic lesions.

In the cases where ureteral involvement is suspected, as the course of the ureters is posteromedial over the external iliac vessels and passes through the paracervical space, lateral to the uterosacral ligaments to reach the meastuses on the bladder, oblique coronal T2W MR images are acquired. These images are obtained paralled to the short axis of the uterus. To assess ureteral meastuses, parasagittal T2W images are used.

Diffusion-Weighted Imaging (DWI), a functional imaging sequence that yields information about water mobility and tissue cellularity may be added to the protocol. This sequence also allows the calculation of the apparent diffusion coefficient (ADC) from images with different b values. ADC value describes water diffusibility and is reduced in the presence of causes that reduce water diffusion. ADC can be used in differentiating malignant from benign lesions. Endometriomas have low ADC values in part because of "T2 blackout effects". On a diffusion-weighted image obtained with a low *b* value (which is a type of T2-weighted fat-suppressed image), an endometrioma exhibits low signal intensity resembling the T2 shading as described previously [20].

SUGGESTED MRI PROTOCOL	
T1W	Axial
T1W FatSat	Axial, Sagittal
T2W	Axial, Coronal, Sagittal
IN OTHER SUSPECTED PATHOLOGY	
T1W Post Gadolinium	Axial, Coronal, Sagittal
Diffusion-weighted imaging	

Table 2. Suggested MRI Protocol

^{18}F-fluorodeoxyglucose positron emission tomography (FDG-PET) scan

The value of ^{18}F-fluorodeoxyglucose positron emission tomography (FDG-PET) uptake in endometriosis has not yet been extensively reported. Most literatures report that majority of endometriomas have low FDG metabolism. Although the exact mechanism is not understood, the endometiomas may show FDG uptake due to inflammation.

Conclusion

Plain radiography, barium enema studies and CT scans are neither sensitive nor specific for the diagnosis of endometriosis.
Ultrasound is the most common imaging modality however it is only useful in the evaluation of endometriotic cysts. It is not sensitive for superficial lesions and detection of adhesions or implants.
MR is the most sensitive and specific imaging technique however it is not sensitive for superficial lesions. MR is accurate in distinguishing endometriomas from other masses. In one study, MRI showed a sensitivity of 90-92% and a specificity of 91-98% for the diagnosis of endometrioma in patients with adnexal masses [21]. In general, comparison studies of ultrasound and MR imaging have shown MR imaging to be better in differentiation of benign from malignant masses on the basis of accurate identification of fat and hemorrhage in benign tumors [22]. False-negative findings are seen in patients with small peritoneal implants, as they are too small to be detected by MR or any other noninvasive imaging. False-positive findings occur because cystic neoplasms and functional cysts can mimic endometriomas.

References:

[1] Woodward PJ, Sohaey R, Mezzetti TP. Endometriosis: radiologic-pathologic correlation. RadioGraphics 2001; 21(1):193-216.

[2] Márcia MC, Ivone Dirk SF, Luciana MPC, Ivete Á, Márcia CFF. Clinical Prediction of Deeply Infiltrating Endometriosis before Surgery: Is It Feasible? A Review of the Literature. Biomed Res Int. 2013; 564.

[3] Del FC, Girometti R, Pittino M, Del FG, Bazzocchi M, Zuiani C. Deep retroperitoneal pelvic endometriosis: MR imaging appearance with laparoscopic correlation. RadioGraphics 2006; 26(6):1705-1718).

[4] Chapron C, Chopin N, Borghese B, et al. Deeply infiltrating endometriosis: pathogenetic implications of the anatomical distribution. Human Reproduction. 2006; 21(7):1839-1845.

[5] Gordon RL, Evers K, Kressel HY, Laufer I, Herlinger H, Thompson JJ. Double-contrast enema in pelvic endometriosis. AJR Am J Roentgenol 1982; 138:549-552.

[6] Patel MD, Feldstein VA, Chen DC, Lipson SD, Filly RA. Endometriomas: diagnostic performance of US. Radiology 1999; 210:739-745.

[7] Ferreira MCF, Carneiro MM. Ultrasonographic aspects of endometriosis. Journal of Endometriosis. 2010; 2(2):47–54.

[8] Hudelist G, Ballard K, English J, et al. Transvaginal sonography versus clinical examination in the preoperative diagnosis of deep infiltrating endometriosis. Ultrasound in Obstetrics and Gynecology. 2011; 37(4):480–487.

[9] Grasso RF, di Giacomo V, Sedati P, et al. Diagnosis of deep infiltrating endometriosis: accuracy of magnetic resonance imaging and transvaginal 3D ultrasonography. Abdominal Imaging. 2010; 35(6):716–725.

[10] Guerriero S, Alcázar JL, Ajossa S, Pilloni M, Melis GB. Three-dimensional sonographic characteristics of deep endometriosis. Journal of Ultrasound in Medicine. 2009; 28(8):1061–1066.

[11] Patel MD, Feldstein VA, Chen DC et-al. Endometriomas: diagnostic performance of US. Radiology. 1999; 210 (3): 739-45.

[12] Buy JN, Ghossain MA, Mark AS, et al. Focal hyperdense areas in endometriomas: a characteristic finding on CT. AJR Am J Roentgenol. Oct 1992; 159(4):769-71.

[13] Bazot M, Darai E, Hourani R et-al. Deep pelvic endometriosis: MR imaging for diagnosis and prediction of extension of disease. Radiology. 2004; 232 (2): 379-89.

[14] Outwater E, Schiebler M L, Owen R S, Schnall M D. Characterization of hemorrhagic adnexal lesions with MR imaging: blinded reader study. Radiology February 1993 Volume 186, Issue 2

[15] Choudhary S, Fasih N, Papadatos D, Surabhi VR. Unusual imaging appearances of endometriosis. AJR Am J Roentgenol 2009; 192(6):1632–1644.

[16] Gougoutas CA, Siegelman ES, Hunt J, Outwater EK. Pelvic endometriosis: various manifestations and MR imaging findings. AJR Am J Roentgenol 2000; 175(2):353–358.

[17] Antônio C, Leonardo KB, Cíntia E P, Flávia J, Cláudio M A, Elisa C, Marisa AD, Romeu CD, Edson M, MR Imaging in Deep Pelvic Endometriosis: A Pictorial Essay. Radiographics March-April 2011 Volume 31, Issue 2.

[18] Siegelman ES, Outwater EK. Tissue characterization in the female pelvis by means of MR imaging. Radiology 1999; 212(1).

[19] Gougoutas CA, Siegelman ES, Hunt J, Outwater EK. Pelvic endometriosis: various manifestations and MR imaging findings. AJR Am J Roentgenol. 2000; 175(2):353-8.

[20] Evan S. Siegelman, Edward R. Oliver, MR Imaging of Endometriosis: Ten Imaging Pearls. Radiographics October 2012 Volume 32, Issue 6.

[21] Togashi K, Nishimura K, Kimura I, et al. Endometrial cysts: diagnosis with MR imaging. Radiology. Jul 1991; 180(1):73-8.

[22] Kurtz AB, Tsimikas JV, Tempany CM, et al. Diagnosis and staging of ovarian cancer: comparative values of Doppler and conventional US, CT, and MR imaging correlated with surgery and histopathologic analysis-- report of the Radiology Diagnostic Oncology Group. Radiology. Jul 1999; 212(1):19-27.

5 PHARMACOTHERAPY OF ENDOMETRIOSIS

Dr Sowmya Sham Kanneppady; MBBS, MD Pharmacology

Faculty of Medicine, Lincoln University College, Malaysia

Endometriosis is a gynecological disorder characterized by presence of endometrial tissues outside the uterus (1). Current treatment modalities are focused on inducing hypo-estrogenic state, as endometriosis is a disease of hyper-estrogenic state. The available treatment modalities suppress the ectopic endometrial tissue, but leaving the risk of recurrence of disease (2, 3). Available treatment for endometriosis is oral contraceptive pills, progestins, gonadotropin releasing hormone analogues and androgenic drugs. The above mentioned treatment modalities cause suppression of ovarian functions causing to hypoestrogenic state which result in regression of ectopic endometrial tissue. These are effectively providing symptomatic relief, but with significant adverse effects which can include delayed conception. As these pharmacological agents are not suitable for women who want to conceive, newer drugs have been introduced that aim at new targets. These include GnRH antagonists, aromatase inhibitors, selective estrogen-receptor modulators, progesterone antagonists, selective progesterone receptor modulators (3).

Classic Pharmacological Approach for Endometriosis:

Non-steroidal anti-inflammatorydrugs (NSAIDS):

The NSAIDs are the most widely used drugs for pain relief in endometriosis. As endometriosis is a chronic inflammatory condition, anti-inflammatory drugs are the first line therapeutic agents for endometriosis-related pain. Naproxen, ibuprofen, mephenamic acid are the commonest NSAIDs used for this purpose.

The NSAIDs target the cyclo-oxygenase (COX) enzyme which helps synthesizing inflammatory mediator prostaglandins. Inhibition of prostaglandin synthesis causes anti-inflammatory and analgesic effects. Cycloxygenase enzyme exists in 2 forms, COX-1 and COX-2. Non selective NSAIDs like naproxen, mephenamic acid inhibit both enzymes leading gastric mucosal damage. Selective COX-2 inhibitors like celecoxib, etoricoxib have less gastric damage and better are tolerated in patients who cannot tolerate non selective NSAIDs. However there is inconclusive evidence to show that NSAIDs are effectively causing pain relief in endometriosis (4). According to Cochrane review 2015, NSAIDs are found to be more effective than paracetamol in pain relief, but superiority of NSAID over other NSAIDs, or superiority of selective COX -2 inhibitors over non selective NSAIDs are not yet established (5). Some NSAIDs in addition to inhibition of the prostaglandin synthesis, act also through the activation of endogenous opioids and serotonergic mechanisms, which can elucidate the efficacy of NSAIDs in chronic pain conditions. Opioids and NSAIDs are combined due to their synergistic effect which may contribute to reduction or even prevention of morphine tolerance and be opiate sparing effect (6). Significant side effects of NSAIDs include gastric ulcerations. Long-term use of NSAIDs can cause renal damage due to capillary necrosis and ultimately renal failure. As prostaglandins are involved in the follicle rupture mechanism at ovulation, it is not recommended to take NSAIDs during the time of ovulation by women who wish to conceive (7).

Table 1: Common NSAIDs used in endometriosis, their dosage and their half-lives.

NSAIDs	Dosage	Plasma half-life ($t_{1/2}$)
Naproxen	250-500mg BD or TDS	12-16 hours
Mephenamic acid	250-500mg TDS	2-4 hours
Ibuprofen	400-600mg TDS	2-4 hours
Diclofenac	50mg TDS	2 hours

Combined oral contraceptives (COC):

Endometriotic lesions regress during pregnancy due to the high levels of progesterone in maternal blood. Remission of endometriosis continues if women are lactating post-partum due to suppression of oestrogen release from ovaries by prolactin. Clinical observation of regression of symptoms and signs of endometriosis during pregnancy and lactation has led to the use of combined oral estrogen and progesterone for the treatment of endometriosis.

Primary mechanism of combined oral contraceptives is to have a negative feedback on pituitary and hypothalamus, thus inhibiting the release of FSH and LH (8, 9). The COCs have the great advantage over other hormonal treatments in that they can be taken indefinitely and is generally more acceptable to women than alternative hormonal therapy, which improves compliance (10).

Administration of COC can be in two ways, continuous and cyclical administration.

1. **Combined oral contraceptives-Continuous/extended administration**

Continuous/extended administration of combined oral contraceptive induces pseudopregnancy like state with prolonged of amenorrhoea. They are available for 91 days, 365 days and also as mini continuous pills for 24 days and 26 days. They have continuous administration of COC with 7 days of placebo pills during that period withdrawal bleeding occurs. With the use of continuous COC withdrawal bleeding is scheduled once in 3 months(91 days regime) or once in 12 months (365 days regime); the resultant prolonged amenorrhoea regresses the endometriotic lesions due to lack of bleeding at endometriotic sites. The most commonly reported side effect with continuous or extended regimen of COC is breakthrough vaginal bleeding (11). The incidence of breakthrough bleeding and spotting is initially high with continuous dosing but appears to decrease consistently over time. Whether amenorrhea rates would continue to increase after one year of treatment is uncertain because no studies have evaluated treatment beyond one year (11-13). When COC containing low dose of estrogens used continuously can be effective in the management of endometriosis (14). According to the systematic review conducted by Zarbas et.al, continuous COC administration without pill free interval following conservative surgery was more beneficial than cyclical administration of COC (15).

Table 2: Extended/continuous regimes and their dosage:

Regimens of extended/contin	Dosage

uous COC

365 regimen	20µg of Ethinylestradiol + 0.09mg levonorgestrel
84/7 regimen (91 days)	30µg of Ethinylestradiol + 0.15mg levonorgestrel
24/4 regimen	20µg of Ethinylestradiol + 3mg of drospirenone
	20µg of Ethinylestradiol + 1mg of norethindrone

2. Combined oral contraceptives-Cyclical administration

Cyclical COC (with estrogen and progestin) are administered for duration of 21 days followed by 7 days pill free or placebo pill period. There are 4 different generations of COCs depending mainly on the type of progestin used and the amount of estrogen/progestins in them. While first generation COC pills are no longer available, Second generation COC pills contain progestin, levonorgestrel and norethisterone are in use. Consequently third generation COC pills containing norgestimate, desogestrel, gestodene and cyproterone acetate are introduced. Fourth generation COC pills contain a progestin drospirenone (16).

The cyclical use of low dose COC ensures reduced menstrual blood flow which benefits the women who have prolonged, frequent menstrual bleeding which is a known endometriosis risk factor. Cyclical low dose COC is well tolerated in many women with fewer side effects compared to GnRH analogues. It was found that COC reduces dyspareunia and non-cyclical pelvic pain. The COC are considered to be first line in the management of endometriosis associated with pelvic pain and can be combined with NSAIDs (17, 18).

Table 3: Cyclical COC and dosage

Cyclical COC	Dosage
Second generation cyclical COC	Ethinylestradiol 30µg +levonorgestrel 150 µg
	Ethinylestradiol 30µg +norethisterone 1.5mg
	Ethinylestradiol 20µg +norethisterone 1mg
Third generation cyclical COC	Ethinylestradiol 35µg +norgestimate 250 µg
	Ethinylestradiol 30µg +desogestrel 150 µg
	Ethinylestradiol 35µg +cyproterone acetate 2mg
Fourth generation cyclical COC	Ethinylestradiol 30µg +drospirenone 3mg

Progestins:

Progestins are synthetic progestogens with functions similar to physiological progesterone hormone. Four recognized generations of progestins have their own advantages and disadvantages. Progestins are safer and cheaper than other hormonal agents like GnRH analogues and danazol. Progestins are available as oral, injectables and intrauterine devices.

Progestins cause decidualization of eutopic and ectopic endometrial tissues which ultimately result in endometrial atrophy. Side effects of progestins include breakthrough bleeding, bloatedness, weight gain and breast tenderness.

Norethisterone acetate (norethindrone acetate) is a progestogen derivative of 19-nortestosterone (19). It has progestational action; apart from that it also has weak androgenic and estrogenic actions at higher doses. Its mechanism of action includes suppression of gonadotropin release, inhibition of ovulation and decidual changes in endometrium. It is available as 2.5-5 mg tablets. Its use for symptomatic and endoscopically confirmed endometriosis has resulted in symptomatic relief from dysmenorrhoea and pelvic pain. (20-22) Efficacy in terms of pain relief is comparable to dienogest (23).

Dienogest is a synthetic progestogen derivative of 19-nortestosterone with anti-androgenic property lacking estrogenic, androgenic property of norethisterone. Dienogest 2 mg/day tablets are available for treatment of endometriosis. Benefit being its lack of androgenic property compared to norethisterone (24, 25).

Medroxyprogesterone is a 17-hydroxy derivative of progesterone displaying androgenic activity and minor impact on the lipoprotein profile (21). Medroxyprogesterone is available as oral tablets (30-60mg/day) and also as depot intramuscular injections (50-150mg IM injections). 50mg depot injection has to be given every week, 100mg injection once in 2 weeks and 150mg injection is to be given every 2-3 months. Medroxyprogesterone in women with symptomatic endometriosis is more efficacious than placebo, and no less efficacious than GnRH agonists, in reducing pain (26). Long acting once in 3 months (150mg) intramuscular injection of medroxyprogesterone acetate has shown risk of reduction in bone mineral density, but this effect being reversible on cessation (27, 28). Depot injections of medroxyprogesterone carry all side effects of progestin and also prolonged amenorrhoea which restricts its use in women who wish to conceive (26). Depot medroxyprogesterone injections for 1 year were compared to the combination of COC and low dose danazol with greater reduction of dysmenorrhoea having higher patient satisfaction. (29)

Levonorgestrel is a potent 19-nortestosterone

derivative, having androgenic and anti-estrogenic effects on the endometrium (30). An intrauterine device releasing 20 mg/day of levonorgestrel induces endometrial atrophy leading to amenorrhea, thus relieving pain and dysmenorrheoa related to endometriosis. This device contains 52 mg of levonorgestrel, which is slowly released into the uterus over a period of up to 5 years. Efficacy of the levonorgestrel intrauterine device is comparable to GnRH analogue in terms endometriosis related pain, with bleeding scores higher in levonorgestrel group (31).

Overall, progestins in any form (oral, injectables and IUCD) has very significant efficacy in terms of reduction in pain related to endometriosis and are considered to be first line agents with fewer tolerable side effects.

Table 4: Types of progestins with examples and dosage (which exerts progestational activity on endometrium with antigonadotrophic activity (32).

Types of Progestins	Examples	Dosage (oral)
17α-hydroxy derivative	Medroxyprogesterone acetate	10mg/day
	Cyproterone acetate	1mg/day
17α-Hydroxynorprogesterone derivatives	nomegestrol	5mg/day
19 Nortestosterone derivatives	Norethisterone	0.5mg/day
	Norgestimate	0.2mg/day
	Levonorgestrel	0.05mg/day
	Desogestrel	1mg/day

	Gestodene	0.03/day
	Dienogest	1mg/day
Spironolactone derivative	Drospirenone	2mg/day

Gonadotropin releasing hormone analogues (GnRHanalogues/agonists):

Pulsatile release of GnRH from hypothalamus leads to stimulation of pituitary for the production and release of FSH/LH. GnRH agonists are longer acting and bind with GnRH receptor for longer period. Initial binding with GnRH receptor causes flare up of release of gonadotrophins. With continuous stimulation of these receptors by GnRH agonists, there is down regulation and desensitization of GnRH receptors leading to reduced levels of gonadotrophins, thus producing hypoestrogenic states and reduction in ovarian activities. Significant adverse effects are related to prolonged hypoestrogenic state which includes hot flushes, headache, and osteoporosis.

GnRH agonists inhibit cell proliferation and increases apoptosis of endometriotic cells (33). Treatment with GnRH agonists is symptomatic, recurrence however occurs after cessation of treatment (34).

They are administered as subcutaneous injections (Goserelin), as nasal spray every 12 hours (naferelin) and leuprolide monthly depot intramuscular injection (leuprolide).

According the Cochrane Database metaanalyses, GnRH agonists are found to be effective in reducing endometriosis-associated pain ,no difference in efficacy between GnRH agonists andother drugs for endometriosis (danazol, COCs, gestrinone) but with much higher adverse effect profiles(35,36). Adverse effects of GnRH analogues are vaginal bleeding, hot flushes, vaginal dryness, decreased libido, breast tenderness, insomnia, and depression/emotional lability. GnRH agonists use cannot exceed the 6 months limit as prolonged exposure reduces bone mineral density leading to osteoporosis (37, 38). According to the Cochrane review, GnRH agonists are although effective in relieving endometriosis related pain (39) they were found to be inferior to the levonorgestrel-releasing intrauterine system or oral danazol. It also concluded that GnRH agonist have significant adverse effects (40). Limited evidence suggests an improvement in quality (41).

Side effects of prolonged therapy of GnRH agonists can be reversed/reduced by use of "add-back" therapy. Add-back therapy aims to effectively treat endometriosis and endometriosis-associated pain, while preventing vasomotor symptoms and bone loss. Add-back therapy includes tibolone 2.5 mg/day which is an estrogen-progesterone mimicking agent (42,43), or by an oestrogen/progestagen combination, i.e. conjugated oestrogens 0.625 mg combined with medroxyprogesterone acetate 2.5 mg (44) or with norethindrone acetate 5 mg (40), oestradiol 2 mg and norethisterone acetate 1 mg (45). "Draw-back therapy" has been suggested as an alternative in a recent study showing that 6 months intake of 400 microgram nafarelin/day was as effective as "draw-back regimen" consisting of 1 month intake of 400 microgram nafarelin/day followed by 5 months 200 microgram nafarelin/day, with similar oestradiol levels (30 pg/mL) but less loss of bone mineral density (46).

Table 5: GnRH analogues and their dosage (47).

GnRH analogues	Dosage	Route of administration
Leuprolide	1mg/day daily	Subcutaneous injection
Leuprolide depot	3.75mg monthly	Intramuscular injection
Triptorelin	3mg	Intramuscular

	monthly	injection
Triptorelin depot	11.25mg 3 monthly	Intramuscular injection
Goserelin	3.6mg	Subcutaneous injection
Buserelin	300-400µg thrice daily	Intranasal
Nafarelin	200-400µg twice daily	intranasal

Table 6: Add back regimen (47).

Regimen	Drugs	Duration
Progesterone only	Medroxyprogesterone	6 months
	Norethindrone acetate	12 months
Progestin +bisphosphonate	Norethindrone + Etidronate	48 weeks
Progestin + estrogen	Medroxyprogesterone + conjugated equine estrogen	6 months
	Medroxyprogesterone + 17β estradiol	6 months
	Norethindrone + 17β	6 months

	estradiol	
	Norethindrone + conjugated equine estradiol	12 onths

Danazol:

Danazol is an androgenic drug with progestational activities. It suppresses ovarian function through a direct inhibitory effect on ovarian steroidogenesis and through inhibition of FSH and LH secretion. Danazol induces pseudomenopause characterized by complete suppression of ovarian function, amenorrhea and hypoestrogenic state. Uterine as well as ectopic endometrium undergoes atrophy during treatment, resulting in a regression and disappearance of endometriosis. Danazol therapy is started with the onset of the menstrual period and should be continued for three to six months or longer depending on the initial extent of the disease and a clinical response (48, 49).

Danazol exhibits some significant side effects due to androgenic properties which includehirsutism, mood changes, weight gain, fluid retention, breast atrophy, voice deepening, and adverse lipid profiles (50,51) It also has hepatotoxicity. Eventhough inexpensive, because of its androgenic side effects, it is less preferred drug for the treatment of endometriosis (19, 52).

Intravaginal danazol is highly effective the treatment of painful symptoms associated with recurrent and deeply infiltrating endometriosis with no systemic side effects (53). The vaginal danazol is a good alternative for repeated surgery and in the treatment of infiltrating endometriosis pelvic pain and adenomyosis (54, 55).

Novel treatment approaches for endometriosis:
1. Aromatse inhibitors:

Aromatase inhibitors are FDA approved drugs for the treatment of ER +ve breast cancer in postmenopausal women. Its effect of causing hypoestrogenic state, rationalizes its use in endometriosis. Aromatase inhibitors inactivates the enzyme which converts androgens to estrogen creating a hypoestrogenic states, thus beneficial in regressing endometriotic lesions.(56) Anastrozole, letrozole are the third generation aromase inhibitors having greater potency and high efficacy with less side effects than the first two generations of aromatase inhibitors(57).

Added advantage of using aromatase inhibitors is, it can treat infertility associated with endometriosis. With the use of aromatase inhibitors, there is initial hypoestrogenic state with consequent increase in the release of gonadotrophins which directly stimulate ovaries. Ovarian Stimulation leads to maturation of ovarian follicle, which enhances chances of conception (58). In premenopausal women who donot wish to conceive, aromatase inhibitors are to be combined with COC or progestins or GnRH analogues to prevent flaring up of gonadotrophins(59, 60). Letrozole is found to be more efficacious in terms of ameliorating endometriosis related pain (61).

Aromatase inhibitors are known to cause side effects due to hypoestrogenic state which includes hot flushes, headaches and accelerated bone loss leading to osteoporosis. Bone loss was found to be reduced if aromatase inhibitors are combined with COC and accelerated bone loss when combined with GnRH agonists for a period of 6 months (62). Exemastane compared to other aromatase inhibitors has bone loss sparing effect (63).

2. GnRH antagonists:

GnRH antagonists like ganirelix, cetrorelix are antagonists at GnRH receptors. By antagonizing GnRH receptors they cause complete suppression of gonodotrophin release without causing initial stimulation (64, 65). Side effects of GnRH antagonists include hot flushes, loss of libido vaginal dryness (66). No conclusive evidence exists for the clear benefit of these classes of drugs for endometriosis (26).

3. Selective estrogen receptor modulators (SERMs):

SERMs are non-steroidal drugs have estrogenic and anti-estrogenic activity in a tissue specific manner. They bind to estrogen receptors (ERs) and can act as estrogen agonists at some tissues and antagonist at other tissues (67).Tamoxifene is FDA approved SERM for the treatment of breast cancer in pre and post-menopausal women due to antagonist action at estrogen receptors in breast carcinoma cells. Raloxifene is an approved drug for prevention and treatment of postmenopausal osteoporosis as it has partial estrogenic receptor agonistic activity at bone. Raloxifene has antagonistic action at endometrial tissue, which makes it an option to use in endometriosis (68, 69). However use of raloxifene has increased risk of adverse effects like hot flushes, leg cramps,vaginal dryness, deep vein thrombosis and pulmonary edema (70-73). Raloxifene has shown to mitigate chronic pelvic pain due to endometriosis (74).Tamoxifene has also been suggested for endometriosis treatment (75). Bazedoxifene is another SERM which has shown to reduce endometriotic lesions in animals by suppressing estrogen induced endometrial proliferations (76, 77).

4. Selective progesterone receptor modulators (SPRMS):

SPRM are novel progesterone receptor ligands with a high degree of endometrial selectivity that exhibit agonist/antagonist impact based on the target tissue, dose and presence or absence of progesterone (78). They cause reversible amenorrhea by selective inhibition of endometrial proliferation with direct effect on endometrial vascularity and have a potential to suppress endometrial prostaglandin production without the side effects of estrogen deprivation (79). Asoprisnil is the first SPRM which is in an advanced stage of clinical development for the treatment of endometriosis. Asoprisnil can suppress both the menstrual cycle and endometrial growth (79). It has found to reduce menstrual and non-menstrual pelvic pain. It has shown safety profile with no hypoestrogenic side effects (80, 81).

5. Antiprogestins:

Mifepristone is a potent antiprogestin with antiglucocorticoids and antiandrogenic property. It prevents progesterone from its action being an antagonist at progesterone receptor.Mifepristone has shown to reduce endometriosis in animal models. Onapristone is another antiprogestin which has found to reduce endometriosis (82). Studies have shown that mifepristone at 50mg/day dose for 3 months has resulted in significant reduction in lesions and pain due to endometriosis (83). Low dose mifepristone (5 mg/day) for 6 months also has shown reduction in pain without affecting endometrial lesions (84). A novel anti progestin, telapristone (Proellex®), was superior than mifepristone with less antiglucocorticoid activity (85, 86).Currently it is undergoing Phase 2 clinical trial for premenopausal symptomatic endometriosis for oral administration with 2 different doses (ClinicalTrials.gov:NCT01728454).

Current Guidelines for the Treatment of Endometriosis

European society of Human Reproduction and Embryology (ESHRE) guidelines on endometriosis management (2013):

Depending upon the strength of supporting evidence (scored from 1++ to 4), recommendations are graded from A-D. The GDG wound write good practice points (GPP) based on clinical expertise, if there is lack of evidence.

Grades of recommendations:

A	Requires at least one randomized controlled trial as part of a body of literature of overall good quality and consistency addressing the specific recommendation. (Evidence levels 1a, 1b).
B	Requires the availability of well controlled clinical studies but no randomized clinical trials on the topic of recommendations. (Evidence levels 2a, 2b, 3).
C	Requires evidence obtained from expert committee reports or opinions and/or clinical experiences of respected authorities. Indicates and absence of directly applicable clinical studies of good quality. (Evidence level 4).
GPP	Recommended best practice based on the clinical experience of the guideline development group.

Hierarchy of evidence:

Level   Evidence

1a	Systematic review and meta-analysis of randomized controlled trials (RCTs)
1b	At least one RCT
2a	At least one well-designed controlled study without randomization
2b	At least one other type of well-designed quasi-experimental study
3	Well-designed, non-experimental, descriptive studies, such as comparative studies, correlation studies or case studies
4	Expert committee reports or opinions and/or clinical experience of respected authorities

Empirical treatment of pain symptoms without a definitive diagnosis:

GPP	Empirical treatment for pain symptoms presumed to be due to endometriosis without a definitive diagnosis includes counselling, adequate analgesia, progestagens, the combined oral contraceptive (COC) and nutritional therapy. It is unclear whether the COC should be taken conventionally, continuously or in tricycle regimen. A GnRH agonist may be taken but this class of drug is more expensive, and associated with more side-effects and concerns about bone density

Treatment of endometriosis-associated pain in confirmed disease:

Non-steroidal anti-inflammatory drugs

A   There is inconclusive evidence to show whether NSAIDs (specifically naproxen) are effective in managing pain caused by endometriosis   Evidence Level 1a

(Allen et al., 2005).

Hormonal treatment

A   Suppression of ovarian function for 6 months reduces endometriosis associated pain. The hormonal drugs investigated - COCs, danazol, gestrinone, medroxyprogesterone, acetate and GnRH agonists - are equally effective but their side-effect and cost profiles differ(Davis et al, 2007; Prentice et al., 1999; Prentice et al., 2000; Selak et al., 2007).   Evidence Level 1a

A   The levonorgestrel intra-uterine system (LNG IUS) reduces endomestriosis associated pain.   Evidence Level 1a

Duration of GnRH agonist treatment

A   Treatment for 3 months with   Evidence

a GnRH agonist may be as effective as 6 months in terms of pain relief (Hornstein et al., 1995). Level 1b

GnRH agonist treatment with 'add-back'

A Treatment for up to 2 years with combined oestrogen and progestagen 'add-back' appears to be effective and safe in terms of pain relief and bone density protection; progestagen only 'add-back' is not protective (Sagsveen et al., 2003). However, careful consideration should be given to the use of GnRH agonists in women who may not have reached their maximum bone density. Evidence Level 1a

Surgical treatment

GPP Depending upon the severity of disease found, ideal practice is to diagnose and remove endometriosis surgically at the same time, provided that pre-operative adequate consent has been obtained (Abbott et al., 2003; Chapron et al., 2003b; Fedele et al., 2004a; Redwine and Wright, 2001).

A	Ablation of endometriotic lesions plus laparoscopic uterine nerve ablation (LUNA) in minimal-moderate disease reduces endometriosis associated pain at 6 months compared to diagnostic laparoscopy; the smallest effect is seen in patients with minimal disease (Jacobson et al., 2001). However, there is no evidence that LUNA is a necessary component (Sutton et al., 2001), and LUNA by itself has no effect on dysmenorrhoea associated with endometriosis (Vercellini et al., 2003a).	Evidence Level 1b
GPP	Endometriosis associated pain can be reduced by removing the entire lesions in severe and deeply infiltrating disease. If a hysterectomy is performed, all visible endometriotic tissue should be removed at the same time (Lefebvre et al., 2002). Bilateral salpingo-oophorectomy may result in improved pain relief and a reduced chance of future surgery (Namnoum et al., 1995).	

Pre-operative treatment

A	Although hormonal therapy prior to surgery improves rAFS scores, there is insufficient evidence of any effect on outcome measures	Evidence Level 1b

such as pain relief (Yap et al., 2004).

Post-operative treatment

A	Compared to surgery alone or surgery plus placebo, post-operative hormonal treatment does not produce a significant reduction in pain recurrence at 12 or 24 months, and has no effect on disease recurrence (Yap et al., 2004).	Evidence Level 1a

The above quoted Cochrane review is based on two studies of 6 months post-operative GnRH agonist treatment, indicating that more research is obviously needed. As endometriosis is a chronic oestrogen-dependent disease, further hormonal treatment is often needed in many women.

In a small RCT, the LNG IUS, inserted after laparoscopic surgery for endometriosis associated pain, significantly reduced the risk of recurrent moderate-severe dysmenorrhoea at 1 year follow-up (Vercellini et al., 2003c).

Hormone replacement therapy

C	Hormone replacement therapy (HRT) is recommended after bilateral oophorectomy in young women given the overall	Evidence Level 4

health benefits and small risk of recurrent disease while taking HRT (Matorras et al., 2002). The ideal regimen is unclear: adding a progestagen after hysterectomy is unnecessary but should protect against the unopposed action of oestrogen on any residual disease. However, the theoretical benefit of avoiding disease reactivation and malignant transformation should be balanced against the increase in breast cancer risk reported to be associated with combined oestrogen and progestagen HRT and tibolone (Beral and Million Women Study Collaborators, 2003).

Treatment of endometriosis-associated infertility in confirmed disease:

Treatment of endometriotic lesions

Hormonal treatment

A	Supression of ovarian function to improve fertility in minimal-mild endometriosis is not effective and should not be offered for this indication alone (Hughes et al., 2007). The published evidence does not comment on more severe disease.	Evidence Level 1a

Post-operative treatment

A	Compared to surgery alone or surgery plus placebo, post-operative hormonal treatment has no effect on pregnancy rates (Yap et al., 2004).	Evidence Level 1a

Assisted reproduction in endometriosis

Intra-uterine insemination

A	Treatment with intra-uterine insemination (IUI) improves fertility in minimal-mild endometriosis: IUI with ovarian stimulation is effective but the role of unstimulated IUI is uncertain (Tummon et al., 1997).	Evidence Level 1b

In vitro fertilization

B	In vitro fertilisation (IVF) is appropriate treatment especially if tubal function is compromised, if there is also male factor infertility, and/or other treatments have failed.	Evidence Level 2b

A	IVF pregnancy rates are lower in patients with endometriosis than in those with tubal infertility (Barnhart et al., 2002).	Evidence Level 1a

The recommendation above is based on a systematic review but the working group noted that endometriosis does not adversely affect pregnancy rates in some large databases (e.g SART and HFEA) (Templeton et al., 1996).

A	Treatment with a GnRH agonist for 3-6 months before IVF or ICSI should be considered in women with endometriosis as it increases the odds of clinical pregnancy fourfold. However the authors of the Cochrane review stressed that the recommendation is based on only one properly randomised study and called for further research, particularly on the mechanism of action (Sallam et al., 2006).	Evidence Level 1b
B	Risk for recurrence is no reason to withhold IVF therapy after surgery for endometriosis stage III or IV since cumulative endometriosis recurrence rates are not increased	Evidence Level 2a

after ovarian hyperstimulation for IVF (D Hooghe et al., 2006).

A	Laparoscopic ovarian cystectomy in patients with unilateral endometriomas between 3 and 6 cm in diameter before IVF/ICSI can decrease ovarian response without improving cycle outcome (Dermirol et al., 2006).	Evidence Level 1b

GPP	Laparoscopic ovarian cystectomy is recommended if an ovarian endometrioma ≥ 4 cm in diameter is present to confirm the diagnosis histologically; reduce the risk of infection; improve access to follicles and possibly improve ovarian response. The woman should be counselled regarding the risks of reduced ovarian function after surgery and the loss of the ovary. The decision should be reconsidered if she has had previous ovarian surgery

Newer drugs under clinical trial:

1. Telapristone: It is an anti-progestin under phase 2 clinical trial for premenopausal symptomatic endometriosis (ClinicalTrials.gov:NCT01728454)
2. ERB-041 (selective estrogen receptor-beta agonist): ERB-041 is a selective estrogen receptor-

beta (ERbeta) agonist which has shown anti-inflammatory activity in preclinical models of arthritis and inflammatory bowel disease. As endometriosis is an inflammatory condition, ERB-041 is under evaluation for an experimentally induced model of endometriosis.ERB-041 and possibly other ERbeta selective agonists may be a useful new approach to treating endometriosis. (ClinicalTrials.gov:NCT00110487)
3. Anti TNF- α: As endometriosis is an inflammatory condition, which is mediated by several cytokines including TNF- α. Drugs like Infliximab, which are anti TNF- α drugs are under evaluation for deep endometriosis pain (ClinicalTrials.gov:NCT00604864).
4. BGS-649: It is newer BGS649 developed as once weekly oral aromatase inhibitor for treatment of obese men with hypogonadotropichypogonadism is under evaluation for moderate to severe Endometriosis Patients (ClinicalTrials.gov:NCT01190475).

5. OBE2109: orally active gonadotropin-releasing hormone (GnRH) antagonist is under, Phase 2b trial to assess it's the Efficacy and Safety in endometriosis related pain (ClinicalTrials.gov:NCT02778399).
6. Elagolix (NBI-56418): It is a highly potent, selective, orally-active, short-duration, non-peptide antagonist of the gonadotropin-releasing hormone receptor is under evaluation for treatment of endometriosis associated pelvic pain (ClinicalTrials.gov:NCT00797225).

Future treatment prospectives:

Endometriosis is a disease with chronic inflammation and one of the etiological bases being autoimmune disorder. Various drugs with antioxidant property and immunosuppressive effects have been suggested for the treatment of endometriosis.

1. **Antioxidant:** omega-3 polyunsaturated fatty acids are found to reduce inflammatory pain related to endometriosis. Omega-3 polyunsaturated fatty acid reduces lipopolysaccharide induced IL-8 and PG E2, thus showing the potential to reduce pelvic pain related to endometriosis (87).
2. **Statins:** Statins are hypolipidemic agents which inhibit HMG-CoA reductase enzyme in the liver. Several drugs from this group have found to reduce endometriotic lesions in experimental animals. They have intrinsic antioxidant property (88).
3. **Anti angiogenic drugs:** Ectopic endometrial implant has shown to possess VEGF and VEGF receptors which is a growth factor for the neoangiogenesis. Various compounds have found to be inhibiting angiogenesis in ectopic endometrial implants.

Dopamine and its agonists like bromocriptinehave found to inhibit VEGF expression, thus preventing angiogenesis in endometriosis.

Bevacizumab is a humanised monoclonal antibody against VEGF –R. It has shown to inhibit endometriosis lesion in murine model. (89)

Romidepsin, a histone deacetylase inhibitor inhibit VEGF gene transcription, down regulating VEGF protein expression, thus preventing angiogenesis. Thus romidepsin is a potential drug for inhibiting angiogenesis in endometriosis (90).

Rapamycin is an immunosuppressants has antiangiogenic effect. It inhibits neovacularization and has induced endometriotic lesion regression in vitro models (91).

As endometriosis is a chronic inflammatory condition, drugs which has anti-inflammatory actions like TNF alpha inhibitors, various cytokine inhibitors can be the target for future therapies.

References:

1. Barbieri RL. Endometriosis 1990 - current treatment approaches. Drugs 1990; 39(4): 502-10.
2. Ferrero S, Abbamonte LH, Anserini P, Remorgida V, RagniN. Future perspectives in the medical treatment of endometriosis.ObstetGynecolSurv 2005; 60:817-2.

3. AboubakrE..Emerging treatment of endometriosis.Middle East Fertility Society Journal 2015; 20: 61-69

4. Allen C, Hopewell S, Prentice A, Non-steroidal anti-inflammatory drugs for pain in women with endometriosis.Cochrane Database Syst Rev. 2005; 19 (4): CD004753.

5. Hanna MH, Elliot KM, Stuart-Taylor ME, Roberts DR, Buggy D, Arthurs GJ. Comparative study of analgesic efficacy and morphine-sparing effect of intramuscular dexketoprofentrometamol with ketoprofen or placebo after major orthopaedic surgery. Br J Clin Pharmacol 2003; 55: 126-133.

6. Duffy DM, Stouffer RL. Follicular administration of a cyclooxygenase inhibitor can prevent oocyte release without alteration of normal luteal function in rhesus monkeys. Hum Reprod 2003; 17: 2825-2831.

7. Marjoribanks J, Ayeleke RO, Farquhar C, Proctor M. Nonsteroidal anti-inflammatory drugs for dysmenorrhoea. Cochrane Database of Systematic Reviews 2015; 7: CD001751.

8. Mishell DR, Kletzky OA, Brenner PF, et al. The effect of contraceptive steroid on hypothalamic-pituitary function. Am J Obstet Gynecol. 1977; 128: 60-74.

9. Kristen Page Wright, Julia V Johnson. Evaluation of extended and continuous use oral contraceptives.TherClin Risk Manag. 2008; 4(5): 905-911.

10. Moamar Al-Jefout. Brief update on endometriosis treatment.Middle East Fertility Society Journal 2011; 16: 167-174.

11. Archer DF, Jensen JT, Johnson JV, et al. Evaluation of a continuous regimen of levonorgestrel/ethinylestradiol: phase 3 study results. Contraception, 2006; 74: 439-45.

12. Miller L, Notter KM. Menstrual reduction with extended use of combination oral contraceptive pills: randomized controlled trial. ObstetGynecol, 2001; 98: 771-8.

13. Kwiecien M, Edelman A, Nichols M, et al. Bleeding patterns andpatient acceptability of standard or continuos dosing regimens ofa low-dose oral contraceptive: a

randomized trial. Contraception 2003; 67: 9-13.

14. Moghissi KS. Medical treatment of endometriosis. ClinObstet Gynecol. 1999 Sep;42(3):620-32. Review.

15. Zorbas, K.A., Economopoulos, K.P. & Vlahos, N.F. Continuous versus cyclic oral contraceptives for the treatment of endometriosis: a systematic review.ArchGynecolObstet 2015; 292: 37.

16. Combined Hormonal Contraceptives: Review of Risk of Thromboembolism. Author: MHRA (2014).

17. Vercellini P, Trespidi L, Colombo A, et al. A gonadotrophin releasing hormone agonist versus a low dose oral contraceptive for pelvic pain associated with endometriosis. FertilSteril 1993; 60:75-79.

18. Colin J. Davisa , Lindsay McMillan.Pain in endometriosis: effectiveness of medical and surgical management.CurrOpinObstetGynecol 2003;15: 507-512.

19. Vercellini P, Somigliana E, Viganò P, Abbiati A, Barbara G,Crosignani PG. Endometriosis: Current Therapies and New Pharmacological Developments. Drugs 2009; 69(6): 649-675.

20. Muneyyirci-Delale O, Karacan M. Effect of norethindrone acetate in the treatment of symptomatic endometriosis. Int J FertilWomens Med 1998; 43: 24-7.

21. Vercellini P, Pietropaolo G, De Giorgi O, Pasin R, ChiodiniA, Crosignani PG. Treatment of symptomatic rectovaginal endometriosis with an estrogen-progestogen combination versus low dose norethindrone acetate. FertilSteril 2005; 84: 1375-87.

22. Ferrero S, Camerini G, Ragni N, Venturini PL, Biscaldi E, Remorgida V. Norethisterone acetate in the treatment of colorectal endometriosis: a pilot study. Hum Reprod 2010; 25(1): 94-100.

23. Moore C, Kohler G, Muller A. The treatment of endometriosis with dienogest. Drugs Today 1999; 35 (Suppl C): 41-52.

24. Muneyyirci-Delale O, Karacan M. Effect of norethindrone acetate in the treatment of symptomatic endometriosis. Int J FertilWomens Med 1998; 43: 24-7.

25. Cosson M, Querleu D, Donnez J, Madelenat P, Konincks P, Audebert A, Manhes H. Dienogest is as effective as triptorelin in the treatment of endometriosis after laparoscopic surgery: results of a prospective, multicenter, randomized study. FertilSteril 2002; 77(4):684-692.

26. Sardeli C, AngelosDaniilidis, Goulas A, Papazisis G, Kouvelas D, Tzafettas J. Endometriosis: The Role of Pharmacotherapy. Current Women's Health Reviews, 2012, 8, 138-149.

27. Clark MK, Sowers MR, Nichols S, Levy B. Bone mineral density changes over two years in first-time users of depot medroxyprogesterone acetate. FertilSteril 2004; 82(6): 1580-6.

28. Cundy T, Cornish J, Evans MC, Roberts H, Reid IR.. Recovery of bone density in women who stop using medroxyprogesterone acetate. BMJ 1994; 308(6923): 247-8.

29. Vercellini P, De Giorgi O, Oldavi S, Cortesi I, Panazza S, Crosignani P. Depot medroxyprogesterone acetate versus an oral contraceptive combined with very-low-dose danazol for long-term treatment of pelvic pain associated with endometriosis. Am J ObstetGynecol 1996; 175: 396-401.

30. Salmi A, Pakarinen P, Peltola AM, Rutanen EM. The effect of intrauterine levonorgestrel use on the expression of C-Jun, oestrogen receptors, progesterone receptors and Ki-67 in human endometrium. Mol Hum Reprod 1998; 4(12): 1110-5.

31. Petta CA, Ferriani RA, Abrao MS, Hassan D, Rosa E Silva JC, Podgaec S, Bahamondes L. Randomized clinical trial of a levonorgestrel-releasing intrauterine system and a depot GnRH analogue for the treatment of chronic pelvic pain in women with endometriosis. Hum Reprod 2005; 20(7): 1993-8.

32. Schindler A.E., Campagnoli C., Druckmann R., Huber J., Pasqualini J.R., Schweppe K.W., Thijssen J.H.H. Classification and pharmacology of progestins. Maturitas 2003; 46 (SUPPL. 1): S7-S16.)

33. Tesone M, Bilotas M, Barañao RI, Meresman G. The role of GnRHanalogs in endometriosis-associated apoptosis and angiogenesis. GynecolObstet Invest 2008; 66 (Suppl 1): 10-8.

34. Waller KG, Shaw RW. Gonadotropin-releasing hormone analogs for the treatment of endometriosis: long-term follow-up. FertilSteril 1993; 59: 511-5.

35. Davis L, Kennedy SS, Moore J, Prentice A. Modern combined oral contraceptives for pain associated with endometriosis. Cochrane Database Syst Rev 2007; (3):CD001019.

36. Prentice A, Deary A, Goldbeck-Wood S, Farquhar CM, Smith S. Gonadotrophin-releasing hormone analogs for pain associated with endometriosis (Review). Cochrane Database Syst Rev 2007; (2): CD000346.

37. Pickersgill A. GnRH agonists and add-back therapy: is there a perfect combination? Br J ObstetGynaecol 1998; 105: 475-85.

38. Bedaiwy M, Casper R. Treatment with leuprolide acetate and hormonal add-back for up to 10 years in stage IV endometriosis patients with chronic pelvic pain. FertilSteril 2006; 86: 220-2.

39. Brown J, Pan A and Hart RJ. Gonadotrophin-releasing hormone analogues for pain associated with endometriosis. Cochrane Database Syst Rev 2010:CD008475.

40. Hornstein MD, Yuzpe AA, Burry KA, Heinrichs LR, Buttram VL, Jr. and Orwoll ES. Prospective randomized double-blind trial of 3 versus 6 months of nafarelin therapy for endometriosis associated pelvic pain. FertilSteril 1995; 63:955–962.

41. Zhao SZ, Kellerman LA, Francisco CA and Wong JM. Impact of nafarelin and leuprolide for endometriosis on quality of life and subjective clinical measures. J Reprod Med 1999; 44:1000-1006.

42. Taskin O, Yalcinoglu AI, Kucuk S, Uryan I, Buhur A, Burak F. Effectiveness of tibolone on hypoestrogenic symptoms induced by goserelin treatment in patients with endometriosis. FertilSteril 1997; 67: 40-45.

43. Lindsay PC, Shaw RW, Bennink HJ, Kicovic P. The effect of add-back treatment with tibolone (Livial) on patients treated with the gonadotropin-releasing hormone agonist triptorelin (Decapeptyl). FertilSteril 1996; 65: 342-348.

44. Friedman AJ, Hornstein MD. Gonadotropin-releasing hormone agonist plus estrogen-progestin "add-back" therapy for endometriosis-related pelvic pain. FertilSteril 1993; 60: 236-241.

45. Franke HR, van de Weijer PH, Pennings TM, van der Mooren MJ. Gonadotropin-releasing hormone agonist plus "add-back" hormone replacement therapy for treatment of endometriosis: a prospective, randomized, placebo-controlled, double-blind trial. FertilSteril 2000; 74: 534-539.

46. Tahara M, Matsuoka T, Yokoi T, Tasaka K, Kurachi H, Murata Y. Treatment of endometriosis with a decreasing dosage of a gonadotropin-releasing hormone agonist (nafarelin): a pilot study with low-dose agonist therapy ("draw-back" therapy). FertilSteril 2000; 73: 799-804.

47. Crosignani P, Olive D, Bergqvist A, Luciano A. Advances in the management of endometriosis: An update for clinicians. Human Reproduction Update. 2005; 12(2):179-189.

48. DmowskiWP.Danazol in the treatment of endometriosis and infertility.ProgClinBiol Res. 1982; 112 Pt B: 167-86.

49. Barbieri R.L., Ryan K.J.Danazol: Endocrine pharmacology and therapeutic applications. American Journal of Obstetrics and Gynecology 1981; 141 (4): 453-463.

50. Henzl MR, Corson SL, Moghissi K, Buttram VC, Berqvist C, Jacobson J. Administration of nasal nafarelin as compared with oral danazol for endometriosis: a multicenter double-blind comparative clinical trial. N Engl J Med 1988; 318(8): 485-9.

51. Fraser IS, Shearman RP, Jansen RP, Sutherland PD. A comparative treatment trial of endometriosis using the gonadotrophin releasing hormone agonist, nafarelin, and the synthetic steroid, danazol. Aust N Z J ObstetGynaecol 1991; 31(2): 158-63.

52. Rotondi M, Labriola D, Rotondi M, et al. Depot leuprorelin acetate versus danazol in the treatment of infertile women with symptomatic endometriosis. Eur J GynaecolOncol 2002; 23: 523-6.

53. Razzi S., Luisi S., Calonaci F. et al. Efficacy of vaginal danazol treatment in women with recurrent deeply infiltrating endometriosis. Fertil. Steril 2007; 88: 789-94.

54. Luisi S., Razzi S., Lazzeri L. et al. Efficacy of vaginal danazol treatment in women with menorrhagia during fertile age. Fertil. Steril. 2009; 92: 1351-4.

55. S. Luisi, C. Regini, F. Vellucci, C. Orlandini, S. Razzi, F. Petraglia. New trends in pharmacological treatments of endometriosis. Archives of Perinatal Medicine 2004; 20(2): 69-72.
56. Zeitoun KM, Bulun SE. Aromatase: a key molecule in the pathophysiology of endometriosis and a therapeutic target. FertilSteril 1999; 72:961-9.
57. Oktay K, Hourvitz A, Sahin G, Oktem O, Safro B, Cil A, Bang H. Letrozole reduces estrogen and gonadotropin exposure in women with breast cancer undergoing ovarian stimulation before chemotherapy. J ClinEndocrinolMetab 2006; 91:3885-90.
58. Mitwally MF, Casper RF. Use of an aromatase inhibitor for induction of ovulation in patients with an inadequate response to clomiphene citrate. FertilSteril 2001; 75:305-92.
59. Ailawadi RK, Jobanputra S, Kataria M, Gurates B, Bulun SE. Treatment of endometriosis and chronic pelvic pain with letrozole and norethindrone acetate: a pilot study. FertilSteril 2004;81:290-6.
60. Shippen ER, West Jr WJ. Successful treatment of severe endometriosis in two premenopausal women with an Aromatase inhibitor. FertilSteril 2004; 81:1395-8.
61. Mousa NA, Bedaiwy MA, Casper RF. Aromatase inhibitors in the treatment of severe endometriosis. ObstetGynecol 2007; 109:1421-3.
62. Soysal S, Soysal M, Ozer S, et al. The effects of post-surgical administration of goserelin plus anastrozole compared to goserelin alone in patients with severe endometriosis: a prospective randomized trial. Hum Reprod 2004; 19:160-7.
63. Mousa NA, Bedaiwy MA, Casper RF. Aromatase inhibitors in the treatment of

severe endometriosis. ObstetGynecol 2007; 109:1421-3.
64. Reissmann T, Schally AV, Bouchard P, Riethmiiller H, Engel J. The LHRH antagonist cetrorelix: a review. Hum Reprod Update 2000; 6(4): 322-31
65. Huirne JA, Lambalk CB. Gonadotropin-releasing-hormonereceptor antagonists. Lancet 2001; 358(9295): 1793-803.
66. Küpker W, Felberbaum RE, Krapp M, Schill T, Malik E, Diedrich K. Use of GnRH antagonists in the treatment of endometriosis.Reprod Biomed Online 2002; 5(1): 12-6.
67. Vogelvang TE, van der Mooren MJ, Mijatovic V, Kenemans P. Emerging selective estrogen receptor modulators: special focus on effects on coronary heart disease in postmenopausal women. Drugs 2006; 66:191-221.
68. Stratton P, Sinaii N, Segars J, Koziol D, Wesley R, Zimmer C, et al. Return of chronic pelvic pain from endometriosis after raloxifene treatment: A randomized controlled trial. Obstetrics and Gynecology 2008 January; 111(1):88-96.
69. Eng-Wong J, Zujewski JA. Raloxifene and its role in breast cancer prevention. Expert Review of Anticancer Therapy2004; 4:523-32
70. Francucci CM, Romagni P, Boscaro M. Raloxifene: bone and cardiovascular effects. Journal of Endocrinological Investigation 2005; 28(10 Suppl):85-90.
71. Scott JA, da Camara CC, Early JE. Raloxifene: A selective estrogen receptor modulator. American Family Physician1990; 60:1131-9.
72. Silfen SL, Ciaccia AV, Bryant HU. Selective estrogen receptor modulators: tissue

selectivity and differential uterine effects. Climacteric 1999; 2:268-83.
73. Thiebaud D, Secrest RJ. Selective estrogen receptor modulators: mechanism of action and clinical experience. Focus on raloxifene. Reproduction, Fertility, and Development 2001; 13:331-6.
74. Stratton P, Sinaii N, Segars J, Koziol D, Wesley R, Zimmer C,et al. Return of chronic pelvic pain from endometriosis afterraloxifene treatment: a randomized controlled trial. ObstetGynecol 2008; 111(1):88-96.
75. Haber GM, Behelak YF. Preliminary report on the use of tamoxifen in the treatment of endometriosis. Am J ObstetGynecol 1987;156(3):582-6.
76. Kulak J Jr, Fischer C, Komm B, Taylor HS. Treatment with bazedoxifene, a selective estrogen receptor modulator, causes regression of endometriosis in a mouse model. Kulak J Jr, Fischer C, Komm B, Taylor HS. Endocrinology. 2011; 152(8):3226-32.
77. LyuH , Liu Y , Dang Q ,Chen H ,Chen R . Effect of bazedoxifene on endometriosis in a rat model.Zhonghua Fu Chan KeZaZhi. 2015; 50(4):291-5
78. Chwalisz K, Garg R, Brenner RM, Schubert G, Elger W. Selective progesterone receptor modulators (SPRMs): a noveltherapeutic concept in endometriosis. Ann N Y AcadSci 2002; 955:373-88.
79. DeManno D, Elger W, Garg R, Lee R, Schneider B, Hess- Stumpp H, Schubert G, Chwalisz K. Asoprisnil (J867): a selectiveprogesterone receptor modulator for gynecological therapy. Steroids 2003; 68:1019-32.
80. Chwalisz K, Larsen L, McCrary K, Edmonds A. Effects of the novel selective progesterone receptor modulator (SPRM)

asoprisnil on selected hormonal parameters in subjects with leiomyomata. FertilSteril 2004; 82(Suppl. 2):S306.
81. Chwalisz K, Perez MC, Demanno D, Winkel C, Schubert G, Elger W. Selective progesterone receptor modulator developmentand use in the treatment of leiomyomata and endometriosis. Endocr Rev 2005; 26:423-38.
82. Stoeckermann K, Hegele-Hartung C, Chalisz K. Effects of the progesterone antagonist onapristone (ZK 98 299) and ZK (136 799) on surgically induced endometriosis in intact rats. Hum Reprod 1995; 10:3264-71.
83. Tjaden B, Galetto D, Woodruff JD, et al. Time-related effects of RU486 treatment in experimentally induced endometriosis in the rat. FertilSteril 1993; 59:437-40.
84. Kettel LM, Murphy AA, Mortola JF, et al. Preliminary report on the treatment of endometriosis with low-dose
85. Progesterone antagonists such as cdb-4124 in the treatment of endometriosis, uterine fibroids, dysmenorrhea, breast cancer, etc. US Application Publication
86. Bhaskaran SS, Nair HB. Progestins/Antiprogestins: Role in Pathogenesis and Treatment for Endometriosis. GynecolObstet 2012;2:e105.
87. Novembri R., Luisi S., Carrarelli P. et al. Omega 3 fatty acids counteract IL-8 and prostaglandin E2 secretion induced by TNF-α in cultured endometrial stromal cells. J. Endo. 2011; 3: 34-39.
88. Rocha AL[1], Reis FM, PetragliaF.New trends for the medical treatment of endometriosis.Expert OpinInvestig Drugs. 2012; 21(7):905-19.
89. Ricci AG, Olivares CN, BilotasMA,et al. Effect of vascular endothelial growth factor inhibition on endometrial implant

development in a murine model of endometriosis. ReprodSci 2011; 18(7):614-22

90. Imesch P, Samartzis EP, Schneider M,et al. Inhibition of transcription, expression, and secretion of the vascular epithelial growth factor in human epithelial endometriotic cells by romidepsin. FertilSteril 2011; 95(5):1579-83

91. Laschke MW, Elitzsch A, ScheuerC,et al. Rapamycin induces regression of endometriotic lesions by inhibiting neovascularization and cell proliferation. Br J Pharmacol 2006; 149(2):137-44

6 A REVIEW OF THE MEDICAL TREATMENT OF ENDOMETRIOSIS

Prof Dr Kombara Maheendran; B. Pharm; MBBS; MSc (Clinical Pharmacol.)

Introduction

Endometriosis is characterised by the presence of endometrial tissue on the ovaries, fallopian tubes or other abnormal sites, causing pain and infertility. The disease tends to progress under the repetitive influence of the menstrual cycle. Thus, interrupting or decreasing menstruation is the mainstay of medical therapy. Endometriosis is likely to remain problematic as long as menstruation persists. Fortunately, symptoms can be modulated or alleviated with appropriate treatment.

The dependence of endometriosis on the woman's cyclic production of menstrual cycle hormones provides the basis for medical therapy. Medications currently recommended include gonadotropin-releasing hormone (GnRH) agonists, progestins, oral contraceptive pills, and androgens. Each of these interrupts the normal cyclic production of reproductive hormones. There are some data supporting the use of aromatase inhibitors for refractory or recurrent endometriosis.

Physiology of reproductive hormones:

The male and female hormones of reproduction share significant mechanistic overlap with one another. Androgens, estrogens, and progestins are all steroid hormones that exert their physiologic action by binding to intracellular receptors, then translocating to the nucleus and altering gene transcription. Recent evidence suggests that estrogens may also act on membrane receptors to mediate non-genomic effects.

A. Gonadotrophins:

The gonadotrophs are unique among anterior pituitary gland cells because they secrete two glycoprotein hormones, luteinising hormone (LH) and follicle stimulating hormone (FSH), together referred to as gonadotropins. LH and FSH are both heterodimers composed of α and β subunits. LH and FSH share the same α subunit but possess different β subunit. Gonadotrophs regulate the secretion of FSH and LH independently. The secretion of estrogens, mainly estradiol, requires gonadotropins, luteinizing hormone (LH) and follicle stimulating hormone (FSH). The release of LH and FSH is, in turn, controlled by the hypothalamus, which releases pulses of gonadotropin-releasing hormone (GnRH)

Once secreted, gonadotropins control hormone production by the gonads, promoting the synthesis of androgens and estrogens. Gonadotrophs are then feedback-inhibited by testosterone and estrogen. The effects of estrogen on the anterior pituitary gland are complex. Depending on the rate of change and absolute concentration of estrogen, as well as the stage of the menstrual cycle, both inhibitory and excitatory effects can be produced. Inhibin and activin are two hormones secreted by the ovary that appear to have inhibitory and excitatory effects, respectively, on FSH but not LH secretion.

Peptide GnRH analogues with short half-lives can be administered in a pulsatile way to stimulate a patterned release of gonadotrophin; while analogues with longer half-lives are used to suppress production of sex hormones by desensitising the pituitary gland to the stimulating activity of the releasing factor.

The main pharmacologic difference among the currently approved GnRH analogues is the method of administration. Leuprolide and histrelin are injected once daily; nafarelin is a nasal spray; goserelin is a depot injection administered once per month. Osmotic pump implants are available that deliver leuprolide acetate at a controlled rate for up to 12 months. Long-acting agonists are utilized therapeutically for treatment of several gonadotrophin –dependent conditions, including endometriosis, and uterine fibroids. The main drawback is that gonadotroph suppression does not occur immediately; instead, there is transient increase in sex hormone levels, followed by a lasting suppression of hormone synthesis and secretion.

B. Sex hormones

The synthesis of progestins, androgens and estrogens is closely intertwined. All three groups are steroid hormones derived from the metabolism of cholesterol.

The terminology "progestins, "androgens" and "estrogens" denotes a number of related hormones rather than a single molecule in each group. The progestins consist of progesterone, a common precursor to testosterone and estrogen synthesis. Progestins generally exert antiproliferative effects on the female endometrium by promoting the endometrial lining to secrete rather than proliferate. Estrogens refer to a number of substances that share a common feminizing activity. **17β-Estradiol** is the most potent naturally occurring estrogen, while estrone and estriol are less potent.

All estrogens are derived from the aromatization of precursor androgens. The ovary and placenta most actively synthesize the **aromatase enzyme** that converts androgens to estrogens. Non-reproductive tissues such as adipose tissue, hypothalamic neurons, and muscle can also aromatize androgens to estrogens. After menopause, the majority of circulating estrogen is derived from adipose tissue.

Progestins, androgens and estrogens are all hormones that bind to a related superfamily of nuclear hormone receptors. Once synthesised these hormones diffuse into the plasma, where they bind tightly to carrier proteins such as sex-hormone binding globulin (SHBG) and albumin. Only the unbound fraction of hormone is able to diffuse into cells and bind to an intracellular receptor. Although separate progesterone, androgen, and estrogen receptors exist, complete selectivity of action does not exist because of the close structural similarities among the hormones. Progesterone receptors and androgen receptors are probably derived from a single ancestral receptor. Most progestins have significant cross-reactivity with androgen receptors, and prolonged progestin administration produces an androgenic effect (virilisation).

The progestins, androgens and estrogens are lipophilic steroid hormones that freely diffuse across the plasma membrane into the cytosol of cells. Once inside the cell, the hormone ligand binds to its specific intracellular receptor, which subsequently dimerizes. The dimer then binds to estrogen response elements (EREs) in promoter regions of DNA.

In the ovary, FSH and LH stimulate follicular development and estradiol synthesis by the granulosa cells of the follicle. In the early follicular phase, the low estradiol levels in blood exert a negative feedback effect on FSH, ensuring that only the dominant follicle ripens.

Midway through the cycle, estradiol levels are high and this has a positive feedback effect on LH secretion, leading to the LH surge that causes ovulation. These feedback effects of estradiol are exerted in the hypothalamus, causing a change in the amount of GnRH secreted, and the pituitary gland altering its response to GnRH.

The required follicle develops into the corpus luteum, which secretes estrogen and progesterone until the end of the cycle. During the follicular phase of the cycle, estrogen stimulates endometrial proliferation.

In the luteal phase, increased progesterone release stimulates the maturation and glandular development of the endometrium, which is then shed in the process of menstruation

Hormonal roles in the pathophysiology of endometriosis

Pathophysiologic processes in the reproductive tract involves either disruption of the hypothalamic-pituitary-reproductive axis or inappropriate growth of estrogen-dependent tissue.

Endometriosis is the growth of endometrial tissue outside of the uterus. The fact that endometriosis is usually found in areas surrounding the fallopian tube (ovaries, recto-vaginal pouch, and uterine ligaments) has led to the hypothesis that endometriosis could result from retrograde migration of endometrial tissue via the fallopian tubes during menstruation. Other etiologies are possible, however, including metaplastic tissue growth from the peritoneum, or spread of endometrial cells to extra-uterine sites via lymphatic ducts. There is also evidence of increased aromatase activity in endometrial tissue from such patients. Because foci of endometriosis respond to estrogen stimulation, endometriosis grows and regresses with the menstrual cycle. This can lead to severe pain, abnormal bleeding, and the formation of adhesions in the peritoneal cavity. In turn, adhesions can lead to infertility. Because endometriosis is usually estrogen-dependent, treatment with long half-life GnRH agonists often achieves regression of the disease.

The Medical Treatment of Endometriosis

The dependence of endometriosis on the women's cyclic production of menstrual cycle hormones provide the basis of medical therapy.

The relevant drug classes include modulators of anterior pituitary gland gonadotroph activity and specific antagonists of peripheral hormone action. In addition, sex hormones are often used as replacement therapy or to modify gonadotrophin release. Medical treatment should be reserved for use in patients with pain or dyspareunia, because no pharmacologic method appears to restore fertility

Pharmacologic classes and drugs

Pharmacologic agents have been developed to target most of the steps in gonadal physiology and pathophysiology.

Drugs which are currently used include:

1. Nonsteroidal anti-inflammatory drugs (NSAIDs)

2. Combination oral contraceptives (COCPs)

3. Progestational agents

4. Danazol

5. Gonadotrophin-releasing hormone (GnRH) analogues.

6. Aromatase inhibitors

1. Nonsteroidal anti-inflammatory drugs (NSAIDs)

NSAIDs such as ibuprofen or naproxen are commonly prescribed to help relieve pain and menstrual cramping. These pain-relieving medications have no effect on endometrial implants. However, they do decrease prostarglandin production. Prostaglandins are important inflammatory mediators in the production of pain.

As a definitive diagnosis of endometriosis may take time, NSAIDs are commonly used to control pain. If they are effective in controlling pain, no other procedures or medical treatments are needed. If they do not relieve pain, additional evaluation and treatment are needed.

Non-steroidal anti-inflammatory agents have not been shown to have any benefit in placebo-controlled studies [1].

2. Oral Contraceptive Pills

The development of safe, efficacious contraceptives for women has revolutionized sexual practices. The **two classes** of widely used oral contraceptives are **estrogen/progestin combinations** (OCPs) and **progestin-only** contraceptives.

Combination Estrogen-Progestin Contraceptives(OCPs):

Oral Contraceptive Pills (OCPs) suppress LH and FSH and prevent ovulation. They also have direct effect on endometrial tissues, rendering it compact and thin. The decidualization of endometrial implants, coupled with reduced reflux related to lower menstrual volume, is the mechanism of pain relief of the OCPs.

The estrogen used in combination estrogen-progestin contraceotives is either ethinyl estradiol or mestranol. Use of unopposed estrogens promotes endometrial growth, and early studies of estrogen-dominant contraceptives determined that these agents increase the risk of endometrial cancer. Because of this finding, estrogen is always co-administered with a progestin to limit the extent of endometrial growth.

Numerous progestins are used in estrogen-progestin contraceptives, and all are potent progesterone receptor agonists. Ideally, the progestin would possess activity only at progesterone receptors, but almost all currently available progestins also have some androgenic cross-reactivity. On a molar basis, norgesterol and levonorgesterol have the highest androgenic activity, while norethindrone and norethindrone acetate have lower androgenic activity. The so-called third-generation progestins eg. ethynodiol, norgestimate, etc. have even lower androgen receptor cross-reactivity.

Classical regimens of combination oral contraceptives consist of 21days of drugs followed by 7 days of a placebo pill. The 7-day placebo period removes exogenous hormone stimulation, stimulating the physiologic involution of the corpus luteum that occurs at the end of a normal menstrual cycle.

The lack of estrogen and progestin causes the endometrium to slough, resulting in menstruation. Because the administration of progestin throughout the cycle inhibits the proliferative growth of the endometrium, most women experience lighter menstrual periods when taking combination oral contraceptives, and a women's menstrual cycle often becomes regular.

Women with endometriosis can take OCPs continuously (with no placebos) or cyclically with a week of placebo pills between cycles. The OCPs can be discontinued after 6 to 12 months or be continued indefinitely, depending on patient satisfaction and the desirability of pregnancy. Continuous non-cyclical administration of OCPs for 3 to 4 months helps avoid any menstruation and associated pain.

OCPs act by ovarian suppression and continuous progestin administration. Initially, a trial of continuous or cyclic OCPs should be administered for 3 months. With pain relief, this treatment is continued for 6-12 months. Pregnancy rates following discontinuation of the pill are 40-50%. This applies to a population unselected for stage and fertility status of the disease. Although few choices are available among individual formulations, note that the long-term efficacy of multiphasic preparations remains unproven.

Continuous noncyclical administration of OCPs, omitting the placebo menstrual tablets, for 3-4 months helps avoid any menstruation and associated pain. A study examined a head-to-head comparison of a GnRH analog and continuous oral contraceptives for the treatment of endometrial pelvic pain found both treatments to be equally effective.

Women with endometriosis are at an increased risk of epithelial ovarian cancer [3], and OCPs are believed to protect against this.

3. Progestational agents

In situations where estrogen may be contraindicated, the use of continuous low-dose oral progestins may be warranted. The two progestin-only oral contraceptives are norgesterol and noerethidrone.

Progestin-only OCPs prevent ovulation 70% to 80% of the time, probably because progestins alter the frequency of GnRH pulsing and decrease anterior pituitary gland responsiveness to GnRH

Progestins are similar to combination OCPs in their effects on FSH, LH, and endometrial tissue. They may be associated with more bothersome adverse drug reactions than OCPs; and if a depot (i.e. medroxyprogesterone suspension) is used, return to fertility may be delayed. However, progestins are effective in reducing the symptoms of endometriosis and are also much cheaper than Danazol or GnRH analogues.

Medroxyprogesterone acetate has proven efficacy in pain suppression in both the oral and injectable depot preparations [4, 5]. Oral doses of 10-20mg/d can be administered continuously. The time to resumption of ovulation is longer and variable with depot preparations. Adverse effects include weight gain, fluid retention, depression, and breakthrough bleeding.

Megesterol acetate has been used in doses of 40mg with similar good results [6].

The levonorgesterol- intrauterine system (LNG-IUS) has been shown to reduce endometriosis-associated pain [7]. When inserted at the time of laparascopic surgery, it has been found to reduce the recurrence of dysmenorrhoea by 35% [8].

4. Danazol

Danazol, is an isoxazole derivative of ethisterone with weak progestational, androgenic and glucocorticoid activities. It inhibits the mid-cycle surge of LH and FSH and can prevent the compensatory increase in LH and FSH following castration in animals, but does not significantly lower or suppress basal levels in normal women. Danazol binds to androgen, progesterone, and glucocorticoid receptors and can translocate the androgen receptor into the nucleus to initiate androgen-specific RNA synthesis. It does not bind to intracellular estrogen receptors, but it does bind to sex hormone-binding and corticosteroid globulins.

Danazol is slowly metabolised in humans, having a half-life of over 15 hours. This results in stable circulating levels when it is administered twice daily. It is highly concentrated in the liver, adrenals, and kidneys and is excreted in both feces and urine.

However, it does not inhibit aromatase, the enzyme required for estrogen synthesis. It increases the mean clearance of progesterone and may have similar effects on other active steroid hormones. Ethisterone, a major metabolite of Danazol, has both progestational and mild androgenic effects.

Danazol acts by inhibiting the midcycle follicle-stimulating hormone (FSH) and luteinizing hormone (LH) surges and preventing steroidogenesis in the corpus luteum. It is the most extensively studied agent for endometriosis.

Danazol has been shown to be as effective as any of the newer agents, but with a higher incidence of adverse effects. Its androgenic manifestations include oily skin, acne, weight gain, deepening of the voice, and facial hirsutism. Hypoestrogenic features due to danazol include emotional lability, hot flashes, vaginal dryness, and reversible breast atrophy.

The recommended dose is 600-800 mg/d. However, smaller doses have been used with success. In a small study of 21 patients, vaginal danazol (200 mg/d) was successful in relieving endometriosis-associated pain.

Barrier contraception and estrogen replacement therapy while on danazol therapy

Because of the possibility of virilizing changes in a female fetus, additional barrier contraception must be used while on danazol therapy.

The evidence for estrogen replacement therapy (ERT) in women with postsurgical menopause for treatment of endometriosis is unclear at the present time.

Danazol has been highly effective in relieving the symptoms of endometriosis, but adverse effects may preclude its use. Danazol is a synthetic androgen that inhibits LH and FSH, resulting in a relatively hypoestrogenic state. Endometrial atrophy is the likely mechanism in the relief of pain from endometriosis. Adverse effects related to estrogen deficiency include headache, flushing, sweating and atrophic vaginitis. Androgenic side effects include acne, edema, hirsutism, deepening of the voice, and weight gain.

Danazol should be used with great caution in patients with hepatic dysfunction, since it has been reported to produce mild to moderate hepatocellular damage in some patients, as evidenced by enzyme changes. It is also contraindicated during pregnancy and breast-feeding, as it may cause urogenital abnormalities in the offspring. Because of the possibility of virilizing changes in a female fetus, additional barrier contraception must be used while on danazol therapy.

Danazol has been employed as an inhibitor of gonadal function and has found its major use in the treatment of endometriosis. Danazol therapy should be started when the patient is menstruating. The initial dosage should be 800mg/d, given in two divided oral doses, but this dosage can be titrated down as long as amenorrhea persists and pain symptoms are controlled. Patients with less severe symptoms may be given 200 to 400mg per day, in two divided oral doses. Treatment duration is six months but can be extended to nine months in responsive patients with severe disease. The overall response rate is 84 to 92%, with beneficial effects lasting up to six months after treatment is stopped [9, 10].

5. Gonadotrophin-releasing hormone (GnRH) agonists

GnRH is a decapeptide found in all mammals. Synthetic analogs include goserelin and leuprolide. They are more potent and longer acting than native GnRH or gonadorelin.

Gonadotrophin-releasing hormone is secreted by neurons in the hypothalamus. It travels through the hypothalamic-pituitary venous portal plexus to the anterior pituitary, where it binds to G protein-coupled receptors on the plasma membranes of gonadotroph cells. Pulsatile GnRH secretion is required to stimulate the gonadotroph cell to produce and release LH and FSH.

Sustained nonpulsatile administration of GnRH or GnRH analogs inhibits the release of FSH and LHby the pituitary in both women and men, resulting in hypogonadism.

GnRH agonists produce a hypogonadotrophic-hypogonadic state by down regulation of the pituitary gland. Goserelin and leuprolide are the commonly used agonists.

These drugs inhibit the secretion of gonadotrophin and are comparable to Danazol in relieving pain. Winkel et al., [11], have claimed that GnRH therapy may lead to improvement in pain associated with endometriosis in 85 – 100% women. Furthermore, the pain relief is believed to persist for 6 – 12 months after cessation of treatment.

Like Danazol, GnRH agonists are contraindicated in pregnancy and have hypoestrogenic side effects. In particular, they have been shown to produce a mild degree of bone loss, although this condition reverses after the medication is discontinued. Because of concerns about osteopenia, "add-back" therapy with low dose estrogen has been recommended.

Efficacy of these drugs is limited to pain suppression, and fertility rates may show no improvement [12]. The pain relief is believed to persist for 6 to 12 months after cessation of treatment.

Add-back therapy while on GnRH treatment

Add-back therapy has been shown to prevent loss in bone density and to relieve vasomotor symptoms without reducing the efficacy of GnRH treatment. GnRH agonists have been used for 12 months with norethindrone add-back therapy with good results [13]. Other drugs such as progestins, tibolone maleate and bisphosphonates have also been shown to be useful.

Add-back therapy and empiric therapy

Much interest has been shown in whether estrogen/progestin "add-back" therapy should be instituted to prevent osteoporosis and hypoestrogenic symptoms. Hormone replacement therapy preparations, progestins, tibolone maleate, and bisphosphonates have all been shown to be effective [15, 16]. Add-back therapy has been shown to prevent loss in bone density and to relieve vasomotor symptoms without reducing the efficacy of GnRH regimens. GnRH agonists have been used for 12 months with norethindrone add-back therapy with good results.

A clinical trial has shown that a 3-month empiric course of GnRH, based on a diagnostic algorithm without definitive laparoscopic diagnosis, is efficacious. However, long-term effects of GnRH analogues on bone density in this population remain unproven. Therefore, add-back therapy remains the standard of care while the patient is on GnRH treatment. GnRH therapy has also been proven to relieve the pain and bleeding associated with extrapelvic distant endometriosis [17].

GnRH analogues vs danazol

A Cochrane review comparing GnRH analogues with danazol treatment showed no difference in improvement of dysmenorrhea, dyspareunia, pelvic pain, or pelvic tenderness [18]. Likewise, no difference in retrospective American Fertility Society (rRAFS) score was found at approximately 24 weeks' follow-up. In contrast, studies that evaluated total pain resolution showed greater benefit from GnRH analogues compared with danazol. Side-effect profiles differed, with greater frequency of hot flushes and vaginal dryness with GnRH analogues, whereas danazol treatment resulted in a greater frequency of weight gain, acne, and headaches.

6. Aromatase inhibitors:

A newer approach to the treatment of endometriosis has involved the administration of drugs known as aromatase inhibitors such as **anastrazole** and **letrozole.** These drugs act by interrupting local estrogen formation within the endometriosis implants themselves. They also inhibit estrogen production in the ovary, brain, and other sources.

Aromatase is believed to increase the prostaglandin E levels via increase in the cyclooxygenase-2 (COX-2) expression.

Aromatase inhibitors cause significant bone loss with prolonged use and therefore cannot be used alone. It is best to combine them with GnRH agonists or combination oral contraceptives.

In a systematic review, they were shown to have promising results for pain relief when combined with either progestins, OCPs, or GnRH analogues.[2] However, the authors concluded that the strength of this inference was limited due to lack of sizeable trials.

Summary

In conclusion, medical treatment of minimal or mild endometriosis has not been shown to increase pregnancy rates. Moderate to severe endometriosis should be treated surgically.

Medical treatment should be reserved for use in patients with pain or dyspareunia, because no pharmacologic method appears to restore fertility. Thus, combination oral contraceptives (COCPs), danazol, progestational agents, and gonadotrophin-releasing hormone (GnRH) analogues form the mainstay of medical therapy. All these treatments have similar clinical efficacy in terms of reduction in pain-related symptoms.

Some authorities believe that endometriosis should be suppressed prophylactically by continuous combined oral contraceptives, GnRH analogs, medroxyprogesterone, or danazol in order to cause regression of asymptomatic disease and enhance subsequent fertility. Peritubal and periovarian adhesions can interfere mechanically with ovum transport and contribute to subfertility.

References:

[1] Allen C, Hopewell S, Prentice A, Gregory D. Nonsteroidal anti-inflammatory drugs for pain in women with endometriosis. Cochrane Database Syst Rev. Apr 15

2009: CD004753.

[2] Nawathe A, Patwardhan S, Yates D, Harrison GR, Khan KS. Systematic review of the effects of aromatase inhibitors on pain associated with endometriosis. BJOG. Jun 2008; 115(7): 818-22.

[3] Modugno F, Ness RB, Allen GO, Schildkraut JM, Davis FG, Goodman MT. Oral contraceptive use, reproductive history, and risk of epithelial ovarian cancer in women with and without endometriosis. Am J Obstet Gynecol. Sep 2004; 191(3): 733-40.

[4] Hull ME, Moghissi KS, Magyar DF, Hayes MF. Comparison of different treatment modalities of endometriosis in infertile women. Fertil Steril. Jan 1987; 47(1) 40-4.

[5] Kauppila A. Changing concepts of medical treatment of endometriosis. Acta Obstet Gynecol Scand. July 1993; 72(5):324-36.

[6] Schlaff WD, Dugoff L, Damewood MD, Rock JA. Megesterol acetate for treatment of endometriosis. Obstet Gynecol. Apr 1990; 75(4):646-8.

[7] Varma R, Sinha D, Gupta JK. Non-contraceptive uses of levonorgesterol-releasing hormone system (LNG-IUS)- a systematic enquiry and overview. Eur J Obstet Gynecol Reprod Biol. Mar 1 2006; 125(1):9-28.

[8] Anpalagan A, Condous G. Is there a role for the use of levonorgesterol intrauterine system in women with chronic pelvic pain? J Minim Invasive Gynecol. Nov-Dec 2008; 15(6):663-6.

[9] Dmoswski WP, Kapetanakis E, Scommegna A. Variable effects of danazol on endometriosis at 4 low-dose levels. Obstet Gynecol. Apr 1982; 59(4):408-15.

[10] Razzi S, Luisi S, Calonaci F, Altomare A, Bocchi C, Petraglia F. Efficacy of vaginal danazol treatment in Women with recurrent deeply infiltrating endometriosis. Fertil Steril. Oct 2007; 88(4):789-94.

[11] Winkel CA, Scialli AR. Medical and surgical therapies for pain associated with endometriosis. Womens Health Gend Based Med. Mar 2001; 10(2):137-62.

[12] Surrey ES, Voight B, Fournet N, Judd HL. Prolonged gonadotrophin-releasing hormone agonist treatment of symptomatic endometriosis: the role of cyclic sodium etidronate and low-dose norethindrone "add-back" therapy. Fertil Steril. 1995; 63(4):747-55.

[13] Friedman AJ, Hornstein MD. Gonadotrophin – releasing hormone agonist plus estrogen-progestin "add-back" therapy for endometriosis-related pelvic pain. Fertil Steril. Aug 1993:60(2):236-41.

[14] Caroline Wellberry. Diagnosis and treatment of Endometriosis: Algorithm for treating endometriosis. Am Fam Physician. Oct 1999; 60(6): 1753-1762

[15] Lane N, Baptista J, Snow-Harter C. Bone mineral density of the lumbar spine in endometriosis subjectscompared to an age-similar control population. J Clin Endocrinol Metab. Feb 1991; 72(2): 510-14.

[16] Surrey E, Hornstein M. Prolonged GnRH agonist add back therapy for symptomatic endometriosis patients: Long-term follow-up of a 12-month clinical trial. Fertil steril. 1999; 72:S80.

[17] Brown J, Pan A, Hart RJ. Gonadotrophin-releasing hormone analogues for pain associated with endometriosis. Cochrane Database Syst Rev. Dec 8, 2010; CD008475.

[18] Telimaa S, Puolakka J, Kaupilla A. Placebo-controlled comparison of danazol and high-dose medroxyprogesterone acetate in the treatment of endometriosis. Gynecol Endocrinol. Mar 1987; 1(1):13-23.

7 PSYCHOSOCIAL ASPECTS OF ENDOMETRIOSIS AND CURRENT CONCEPT OF ITS MANAGEMENT

Associate Professor Dr. Suthahar Ariaratnam; M.MED (Psych);

Discipline of Psychological and Behavioural Medicine,

Faculty of Medicine, Universiti Teknologi MARA, Malaysia.

Introduction

Endometriosis was first described by von Rokitansky in the year 1860 [1]. It is one of the most common gynecological condition [2], in which cells from the lining of the uterus (endometrium) appear and flourish outside the uterine cavity [3]. An estimated 10% of women in reproductive age group are affected by this disease [4]. Symptoms of endometriosis are mainly chronic pelvic pain and infertility [5]. As of now there is no cure for this condition. Nevertheless, it can be treated in a variety of ways, including pain medication, hormonal treatments and surgery [6].

However, there is a tendency to inadvertently underestimate the psychosocial management and its implication on the affected women.

Psychosocial manifestations

This chronic conditon has certainly a significant social and psychological impact [7]. Infact the American Society for reproductive medicine has cautioned that a comprehensive assesment to rule out other non gynaegological causes of pelvic pain due to Endometriosis ought to be pursued which include psychological and psychiatric disorders before any definite therapy could commenced [8].

Additionally, it can cause significant emotional pain in several ways. Since the diagnosis can be difficulty, the individual may not be taken seriously if she experienced especially pelvic pain and occasionally this pain may be incorrectly diagnosed as psychological at the onset [9]. This supposed insignificant and sometimes uncaring connotation shown by the doctor or other medical personnel to a woman's pain can be frustrating, depressing and hurtful to the individual. On the other hand, they have also been termed hypochondriac by family members because of their so called perpetual illness [10].

Next is the feeling of shock, anxiety and perhaps depression after being told of the diagnosis for the first time when the individual has been attempting to conceive many years but to no avail. There would be a feeling as though the body has let them down. As a result, it creates feelings of inadequacy or feeling of being less of a woman leading to guilt. This in turn can lower their self esteem as well as self concept.

Moreover, medications that ameliorates symptoms of endometriosis such as gonadotrophin-releasing hormone (GnRH) agonist could on its own induce anxiety and/or depression in these subjects [11, 12]. Indeed Warnock et al [13], in a retrospective pilot study involving 42 female patients and using the Hamilton Depression Rating Scale found that subjects being treated concurrently with an anti-depressant, Sertraline fared significantly better with regards to depressive symptoms compared to the group receiving only GnRH agonist. Consequently, it was inferred that the introduction of anti-depressant was certainly beneficial in the treatment of mood symptoms during the course of GnRH treatment.

Furthermore, because of the intense pain it causes sporadically the disease without a surprise impacts many areas of a woman's life such as time off work, time away from the family, inability to care for children periodically, painful sex, abdominal pain, heavy bleeding, premenstrual tension, inability to attend social activities or participate in sport etc. Consequently, it can make woman feel less in control of their lives, create self-doubt, impacting relationship and can take away their sense of self worth [9, 14, 15, 16]. Besides, the degree of pain stated by patients is frequently not related with disease severity, giving an impression that, other factors are operating namely psychosocial issues [17].

Lorencatto et al, [18], found that the prevalence of depressive symptoms was high at 92% among 50 women aged 24 to 48 years of age with endometriosis and referring pelvic pain.

Kumar et al, [19] using the Structured Clinical Interview for DSM-IV Axis I Disorders revealed that a significantly higher percentage of women in the endometriosis group were found to have bipolar disorder and a poorer quality of life (QoL) than women with pelvic pain not related to the disease.

In study hailing from Brazil [20], which was prospective in design involving 104 women who were having pelvic endometriosis, 86.5% and 87.5% presented with depressive and anxiety symptoms respectively. This study further elucidated that the Quality of Life (QoL) was determined to be below par.

Exploring immune function, stress and endometriosis, it was found that psychosocial domains in this disease was comparable to other chronic pain syndromes [5]. The authors further showed that psychosocial factors such as stress perception and QoL were impaired in infertile women who additionally endured from endometriosis. This psychoemotional changes as described by the authors was so prominent that it had reached the levels of depression.

As elucidated previously, all the abovementioned issues could ultimately lead to reduction in QoL [20].

A systemic review by Jia et al [21], deduced that pain was a convincing indicator of poor Health Related QoL (HRQoL) among individuals with endometriosis.

Moreover, Fourquet et al [22], examining 193 women from Puerto Rico revealed that Endometriosis symptoms like chronic, incapacitating pelvic pain and infertility had negatively and substantially affected the physical and mental health status, HRQoL and productivity at work of subjects with endometriosis. A similar finding was inferred in a review paper by Szpak and colleagues [23].

In summary, as posited by Bitzer [24], there were 6 areas of challenges and stressors endured by patients with endometriosis which are as follows:

1. often the diagnosis is delayed
2. the cause of the disease is unknown
3. it is a chronic recurrent disease
4. it affects young women
5. it is accompanied by chronic pain and dyspareunia
6. it may lead to infertility

He further emphasized that these characteristics entails greater psychological thrust or focus for these patients which could be achieved with an integrated and comprehensive care. As a result, attributes such as respect and empathy, patient centered communication, sufficient response to negative emotions, development of a helpful and lasting therapeutic relationship, psychoeducation, empowerment and shared decision making should be incorporated in this care.

On the contrary, Eriksen et al [17], examined the psychological profile including anxiety and depression in 96 participants from the Department of Gynaecology and Obstetrics at the Odense University Hospital and was unable to confirm previous findings of pain associated with endometriosis that was correlated with increased level of the 2 conditions mentioned.

In another contradictory results by Low et al [15], who revealed an increased level of neuroticism, anxiety and psychaitric morbidity minus depression in subjects with endometriosis as opposed to healthy women. Conversely, another study showed increased levels of depression in individuals with pain that to both healthy controls and women with asymptomatics endometriosis but no diferences in anxiety between the groups [25].

Despite these controversies, literature generally provides support for the increased prevalence of psychiatric manifestation in subjects with endometriosis.

Management

There is certainly a need for designated time for intimate relationships especially when symptoms are least which mean that these relationships engenders more planned rather than spontaneous activity. Planning these social times is very crucial for relationships and to help partner feel loved and needed during these difficult times. Communication between spouse or partners is not only vital but also as it helps them to understand. Accordingly, it also reduces feelings of being unloved or less desired when it is the disease process not the person that is usually responsible for lack of intimacy.

Women often find that they do not always have the energy to cope with their children and do the things for them they used to or want to. Finding ways of streamlining the family activities may be necessary to make the most of the times when symptoms are most tolerable, leaving rest time when they are not. They need to understand that requesting for help is not a sign of weakness but necessary to help her during the difficult times of enduring symptoms. Encouraging children to help will assist the woman herself and allows the family to feel helpful and proactive in her care.Thus, overcoming these issues not only take time but also they may not be resolved over night.

Work issues can be another area of complexity. If woman are able to relate to their superior regarding their condition then there is more scope for understanding if deadlines are not met or regular sick leave is taken. Unfortunately, if woman are not able to do this then it may put more pressure leading to feeling anxious on them in the workplace and thus aggravating the condition further.

Also researching about the disease and educating key people in the woman's life is crucial since together they can comprehend what is happening, thereby reducing possible uncertainty, worry and anxiety.

Reassurance is needed for spouse or partners that whatever the symptoms, they are not imagined or created to excuse behaviour but they are in fact real.

The need to cope using strategies that have been associated with better psychological adjustment such as active coping and positive reinterpretation. While endometriosis can have psychological consequences and those suffering will undoubtedly benefit from psychotherapy to learn effective coping techniques.

Both approaches of reducing stress and engaging adaptive coping styles as mentioned above should be developed besides using the somatic therapy of endometriosis to end the vicious circle of stress, alerted immune system, depression and reduced QoL. This may be achieved by certain relaxing techniques like Jacobson's Progressive Muscle Relaxation [26].

In addition, progressive muscle relaxation which is a systematic approach to attain deep sate of relaxation has been consistently shown to reduce anxiety, depression and QoL in both psychiatric and medical disorders [27, 28, 29]. Besides, its superiority was also demonstarted among endometriosis individuals undergoing GnRH agonist therapy as it was effective in improving anxiety, depression and QoL [30]. Essentially, relaxation technique was shown to have the best evidence of effectiveness when compared to other forms of complementary and self-help treatments to manage anxiety disorders [31]. Whilst some limited evidence exist to establish the efectiveness of relaxation therapy in the treatment of depressive disorder(Jorm et al 2002) [32].

Providing stress management techniques would be undoubtedly another valuable mnagement tool as it useful in circumventing the vicious cycle of inflammation, depression, pain perception, sickness behaviour and stress [33]. Regretably, this is not routinely done or to make matter worst, undervalued in earlier studies [34].

Additionally, referral to a psychologist would be necessary for them to work through relationships, work or other issues, and give strategies to help them cope as mentioned above.

Moreover, the organization of affected women in self support groups [5], has been found to be helpful.

Apart from the basic care which can be easily provided by each treating physician or nurse, some conditions need more specialized care in the context of a multidisciplinary team. These are chronic pain services, Infertility treatment teams, Sexual counselling and therapy and treatment of psychiatric comorbities or sequelae of the disease like depression, anxiety disorder etc. Occasionally referral to a sexual counsellor is necessary to help retrain tired pelvic muscles from years of pain and learnt behaviour from the pain that intercourse can be pleasurable again.

In short a biopsychosocial approach [35], is prudent for the management of these individual as was proposed by psychiatrist George L. Engel way back in 1977. This model emphasizes the importance of interplay between biological, psychological (which entails thoughts, emotions and behaviors), and social (socio-economical, socio-environmental and cultural) components in human functioning in the context of disease or healing [36, 37,

38]. On this premise the biological domain seeks to understand how the cause of the illness stems from the functioning of the individual's body. The psychological factors explores the potential psychological causes for a health problem such as lack of self-control, emotional turmoil, and negative thinking. The social part examines how different social factors such as socioeconomic status, culture, poverty, technology and religion could impact health. Hence, it is imperative that the management of individuals with endometriosis should adopt a broader and integarted approach as provided by the biopsychosocial model than the traditional biomedical model so that these individuals receive not only holistic but also comprehensive care.

Clearly, biopsychosocial care should be integrated into the biomedical diagnosis and therapy of patints with endometriosis so that these patient would eventually receive optimal care.

Conclusion

Indeed in a recent review [39], it was reiterated that aspect of mental health issues in the gynecological situation are not uncommon. Alas, they are often undetected and untreated, and may influence not only the presentation but also management outcomes of the physical condition itself. The review further stated that the prevalent conditions are anxiety and depression which were significantly associated with morbidity especially in the form of impairments in social, occupational and other areas of functioning. Thus, there must be a greater focus on mental health issues of gyanaecological disease including endometriosis.

Accordingly, it is only prudent to evaluate endometriosis from a biopsychosocial perspective [18, 20], so that these individual would receive holistic and eventually optimized care particularly in the minimisation of functionally injury and scarring induced by this progressive disease.

To re-emphasize, endometriosis has a significant impact on both social and psychological in addition to its physical domains. There is an urgent need to develop, explore and evaluate more interventions psychosocially for both women, partners and family living with this chronic and often debilitating state.

References

[1] Rokitansky K. Über Uterusdrüsen-Neubildung. Z Gesellschaft Aerzte (Wien) 1860; 16:577–581.

[2] Spaczynsky RZ & Duleba AJ. Diagnosis of endometriosis. Semin Reprod Med 2003;21:193-208.

[3] Kennedy S, Bergqvist A, Chapron C, D'Hooghe T, Dunselman G, Greb R, Hummelshoj L, Prentice A, Saridogan E. ESHRE Special Interest Group for Endometriosis and Endometrium Guideline Development. ESHRE guideline for the diagnosis and treatment of endometriosis. Hum Reprod 2005; 20:2698–2704.

[4] Eskenazi B, Warner ML: Epidemiology of endometriosis. Obstet Gynecol Clin North Am 1997, 24:235-258.

[5] Siedentopf F, Tariverdian N, Rucke M, Kentenich H, Arck PC. Immune Status, Psychosocial Distress and Reduced Quality of Life in Infertile Patients with Endometriosis. American Journal of Reproductive Immunology; 2008 60(5): 449-461.

[6] "Endometriosis fact sheet". NIH. Retrieved Feb 12, 2013.

[7] Culley L, Law C, Hudson N, Denny E, Mitchell H, Baumgarten M, Raine-Fenning N. "The social and psychological impact of endometriosis on women's lives: A critical narrative review". Human Reproduction Update; 2013; 19 (6): 625–639.

[8] The Practice Committee of the American Society for Reproductive Medicine. Treatment of pelvic pain associated with endometriosis: a committee opinion. Fertility and Sterility 2014; 101:927–935.

[9] Denny E. Women's experience of endometriosis. J Adv Nurs. 2004; 46:641-8.

[10] Cox H, Henderson L, Andersen N, Cagliarini G, Ski C. Focus group study of endometriosis: struggle, loss and the medical merry-go-round. Int J Nurs Pract. 2003; 9:2-9.

[11] Warnock JK, Bundren JC. Anxiety and mood disorders associated with gonadotropin-releasing hormone agonist therapy. Psychopharmacol Bull 1997; 33: 311-316.

[12] Warnock JK, Bundren JC, Morris DW. Depressive symptoms associated with gonadotropin-releasing hormone agonists. Depression & Anxiety 1998a; 7(4):171-7.

[13] Warnock JK, Bundren JC, Morris DW. Sertraline in the Treatment of Depression Associated with Gonadotropin-Releasing Hormone Agonist Therapy. Biological Psychiatry 1998b; 43:464-465.

[14] Lewis DO, Comite F, Mallouh C, Zadunaisky L, Hutchinson-Williams K, Cherksey BD, et al. Bipolar mood disorder and endometriosis: preliminary findings. Am J Psychiatry. 1987; 144:1588-91.

[15] Low WY, Edelmann RJ, Sutton C. A psychological profile of endometriosis patients in comparison to patients with pelvic pain of other origins. Journal of Psychosomatic Research1993; 37(2):111-6.

[16] Jones G, Jenkinson C, Kennedy S. The impact of endometriosis upon quality of life: a qualitative analysis. J Psychosom Obstet Gynaecol. 2004; 25:123-33.

[17] Eriksen HL, Gunnersen KF, Sørensen JA, Munk T, Nielsen T, Knudsen UB Psychological aspects of endometriosis: differences between patients with or without pain on four psychological variables. European

Journal of Obstetrics & Gynecology and Reproductive Biology 2008; 139 :100-105.

[18] Lorencatto C, Vieira MJN, Pinto CLB, Petta CA: Evaluation of the frequency of depression in patients with endometriosis and pelvic pain. Rev Assoc Med Bras 2002; 48: 217-221.

[19] Kumar V, Khan M, Vilos GA, Sharma V. Revisiting the association between endometriosis and bipolar disorder. Journal of Obstetrics & Gynaecology Canada 2011; 33(11):1141-5.

[20] Sepulcri RP, Do Amaral VF. Depressive symptoms, anxiety, and quality of life in women with pelvic endometriosis. European Journal of Obstetrics & Gynecology and Reproductive Biology 2008, 142:53-56.

[21] Jia et al.: Health-related quality of life in women with endometriosis: a systematic review. Journal of Ovarian Research 2012; 5:29.

[22] Fourquet J, Báez L, Figueroa M, R. Iván Iriarte RI, MS, Flores I. Quantification of the Impact of Endometriosis Symptoms on Health Related Quality of Life and Work Productivity. Fertil Steril 2011; 96: 107-112.

[23] Szpak R, Bugala-Szpak J, Drosdzol A, Skrzypulec V. Health-related quality of life in women with endometriosis. Wiadomosci Lekarskie 2009; 62(2):129-34.

[24] Bitzer J. Psychosomatic aspects of endometriosis. Journal of Endometriosis 2011; 3(3):166-170.

[25] Waller KG, Shaw RW. Endometriosis, pelvic pain, and psychological functioning. Fertil Steril 1995; 63 (4): 796-800.

[26] Jacobson E (Ed.), Progressive relaxation, University of Chicago Press, Chicago (1938).

[27] Molassiotis A, Yung HP, Yam BM, Chan FY, Mok TS. The effectiveness of progressive muscle relaxation training in managing chemotherapy-induced nausea and vomiting in Chinese breast cancer patients: a randomized controlled trial. Support Care Cancer 2002; 10: 237-246.

[28] Nickel C, Lahmann C,Muehlbacher M et al.Pregnant women with bronchial asthma benefit from progressive muscle relaxation: a randomized, prospective, controlled trial. Psychother Psychosom 2006; 75: 237-243.

[29] Dehdari T, Heidarnia A, Ramezankhani A, Sadeghian S, Ghofranipour F. Effects of progressive muscle relaxation training on quality of life in anxious patients after coronary artery bypass graft surgery. Indian J Med Res 2009; 129: 603-608.

[30[Zhao L, Wu H, Zhou X, Wang Q, Zhu W, Chen J: Effects of progressive muscular relaxation training on anxiety, depression and quality of life of endometriosis patients under gonadotrophin-releasing hormone agonist therapy. European Journal of Obstetrics & Gynecology and Reproductive Biology 2012; 162(2):211-5.

[31] Jorm AF, Christensen H, Griffiths KM, Parslow RA, Rodgers B, Blewitt KA. Effectiveness of complementary and self-help treatments for anxiety disorders. Med J Aust 2004; (Suppl.7)181: S29-S46.

[32] Jorm AF, Christensen H, Griffiths KM, Rodgers B. Effectiveness of complementary and self-help treatments for depression. Med J Aust 2002; (Suppl.) 176:S84-S96

[33] Watkins LR, Maier SF. The pain of being sick: implications of immune-to-brain communication for understanding pain. Annu Rev Psychol; 2000; 51:29-57.

[34] Tariverdian N, Theoharides TC, Siedentopf F, Gutiérrez G, Jeschke U, Rabinovich GA, Blois SM, Arck PC. Neuroendocrine-immune disequilibrium and

endometriosis: an interdisciplinary approach. Semin Immunopathol. 2007; 29(2): 193-210.

[35] Engel GL. "The need for a new medical model: A challenge for biomedicine". Science 1977; 196 (4286):129-136.

[36] Engel GL: The clinical application of the biopsychosocial model. Am J Psychiatry 1980; 137:535-544.

[37] Engel GL: From biomedical to biopsychosocial: being scientific in the human domain. Psychosomatics 1997; 38:521-528.

[38] Dowling AS. George Engel, M.D. (1913-1999). Am J Psychiatry 2005; 162:2039-2039.

[39] Bryant C, Kleinstauber M, Judd F. Aspects of mental health care in the gynecological setting. Women's Health 2014; 10(3):237-254.

8 ENDOMETRIOSIS AND FUTURE DIRECTIONS

Prof. Dr. Methil Kannan Kutty; FRCPath (London), FRCPA (Australia);

The colossal magnitude of the problem of endometriosis can be best judged from the incidence of endometriosis distressing 5%-15% of women of reproductive age group and equal to 3% -5% of post-menopausal women (Bellelis et al., 2011). Any discussion of futuristic projections for endometriosis will be worthless and academically unethical without allusion to the 'epic' 11th congress of World Association of endometriosis held in France. The workshop at this conference provided an avenue for gynecologists, researchers .educators, reproductive medicine and surgical specialists to discuss diverse issues and challenges faced by them in particular and society of women in general as well as to share the results of their researches and perspectives in their respective fields of interest .The workshop promulgated 56 recommendations for future research in endometriosis. Readers will do well to refer to the admirable, succinct and impactful account presented by (Rogers et al., 2013). The entire proceedings of the conference have been succinctly described with a broad background of the existing knowledge and research on endometriosis with recommendations for future search on areas with voids in the knowledge of facets of endometriosis that await further elucidation or further exploration.. Of note is the accent on research in endometriosis refined by state of the art technologies available currently.

It is appraised that the exorbitant economic burden it imposes economic burden (yearly cost of endometriosis exceeds US $12 000 per woman). Needless to dwell on this cost which imposes a heavy toll on the direct health care and heavier toll on loss of productivity. While admittedly decline of quality of life is a singularly significant forecaster of direct health care total costs and matter very much. Besides, this issue is compounded by the unfortunate inordinate delay, (a mean delay of 6.7 years) between start of symptoms and a surgical diagnosis of endometriosis; each afflicted subject loses on average 10.8 hours of work weekly, mostly attributable to decreased work efficiency. Women with endometriosis face psychological issues that may severely impact their lives.

Ever since the time of the original clinical depiction of endometriosis, much has been achieved in enhancing our understanding of this debilitating disease. Admittedly no one theory of pathogenesis can elucidate all of the defined manifestations of endometriosis, the retrograde menstruation theory is widely acknowledged to account for the dissemination of endometrial cells (Rogers et al., 2013). Burney et al., 2012 emphasized that there is a pressing need for discovering the specific factor or factors that synchronies the persistence and consequent implantation of the displaced endometrium... Intrinsic or acquired properties of the endometrium and flawed immune clearance are areas of interest in elucidating the genesis of endometriotic implants. Clinical and molecular research entails the study of disease heterogeneity, especially in lesional phenotype and histopathologic validation of implants. The changes emblematic of inflammation, estrogen dependence, and progesterone resistance in the pathophysiology of endometriosis-related pain and infertility are fertile fields for dynamic research. Augmented progress in the comprehension of the pathogenesis of this enigmatic disease, preventive strategies, novel non-surgical diagnostic modalities and targeted therapeutics offer great promise for optimistic future. A broad understanding of the histopathogenesis and pathophysiology of endometriosis is of utmost importance for the development of novel diagnostic and treatment approaches for this incapacitating condition (Burney et al., 2012).

There is much scope for research focusing on large scale well controlled clinical studies of women with and without endometriosis as the cause of infertility and pain and women with and without infertility and pain. It is obligatory to ensure participation of control groups in clinical studies and multicenteric randomized trials. (Robert and Hummelsh). The need to extend the genetic studies cannot be overemphasized as currently the techniques are emerging and to make clinical studies available (Paolo Vercellini 2008).

Paolo Vercellini, 2008 proposed that pharmacological management of endometriosis must be set within the framework of long-term therapeutic strategies. Combination of oral contraceptives and progestinsis recommended as the first-line choice, both as a substitute to surgery and as a postoperative adjuvant measure. Medical treatment is not advisable in women in search of conception as reproductive prognosis is not ameliorated (Harmeet Malhotra., 2009).

Administration of TNF binding proteins to block TNF alpha activity, simultaneously as one introduces menstrual endometrium, and then one can substantially impede the development of endometriosis in baboons. Moreover, it is entirely possible to prevent the development of endometriosis-related adhesions (D'Hooghe et al., 2004). Recent advances in the comprehension of pathophysiology of endometriosis, have favored the perception of endometriosis an autoimmune disorder. Thus novel therapies using immunomodulators and other novel compounds are recommended. An ideal drug would be one that treats endometriosis without hampering fertility (Harmeet Malhotra., 2009).

In order to foster and facilitate research into this

devastating disease, a consensus workshop to define future directions for endometriosis research was conducted in conjunction with the epic and memorable 11th World Congress on Endometriosis in September 2011 in Montpellier, France. This workshop aimed to review and update the endometriosis research of priorities consensus statement developed as an aftermath of the 10th World Congress on Endometriosis in 2008 (Bellelis et al., 2011). The monumental and impactful publication by Rogers et al (2013)., expatiating on the background of various facets of endometriosis with existing voids in knowledge and recommendations for research in the respective fields of endometriosis for filling up the gaps should attract the attention of all those interested in endometriosis. There were 56 recommendations for research that have been promulgated, and categorized under 6 subheadings: (a) diagnosis, (b) classification diagnosis, (c) clinical trials, treatment, and outcomes, (d) epidemiology, (e) pathophysiology, and (f) research policy. It is hoped that this consensus international research priorities "blue print" of the workshop participants and researchers will be empowered and encouraged to develop new interdisciplinary research proposals that will also enhance funding support for research on endometriosis.

According to D'Hooghe et al, 2004, future research in endometriosis must concentrate on pathogenetic studies in the baboon model and on the early interfaces between endometrial and peritoneal cells in the pelvic cavity during menstruation. Further Proteomic and genomic methodologies are mandatory to identify prospective distinctions between eutopic endometrium and myometrium in patients with and without endometriosis. Immunomodulatory drugs hampering endometriosis-linked pelvic inflammation may open up novel therapies in the future for endometriosis (D'Hooghe et al 2004).

Recent years have witnessed rapid strides in Proteomic and genomic strategies. As a corollary to this it is essential for further research in Metabolemics including lipidomics in endometriosis to enhance our comprehension of the pathogenesis of endometriosis. The study by Fowler et al 2007 revealed the presence of dysregulated proteins in women with endometriosis comprising: (i) molecular chaperones including heat shock protein 90 and annexin A2, (ii) proteins implicated in cellular redox state, such as peroxiredoxin 2, (iii) proteins involved in protein and DNA formation/breakdown, including ribonucleoside-diphosphatereductase, prohibitin and prolyl 4-hydroxylase, and (iv) secreted proteins, such as apolipoprotein A1. The functions of these proteins suggest their possible role in the pathogenesis of endometriosis. Fowler et al 2007 recommended the utilization of these techniques combined 2-DE gel analysis and mass spectroscopic protein identification on a greater scale to discover endometriosis-linked proteins, thus enhancing the understanding of this multifaceted disease (Fowler et al., 2007).

Although Rasheed et al., 2010 have proven the presence of Endometriosis inducing factor it is vital to extend the quest of its molecular structure which may shed more light on the exact mechanism of its action .Again from therapeutic point of view, discovery of anti endometriosis inducing factor /factors may help prevent the development of endometriosis (Rasheed et al., 2010).

Ishii K et al., 2003 surveyed and compared the prevalence of HLA DQB1 and DPB1 allele frequencies in 83 patients and 222 controls. The study revealed that the incidence of the HLA-DQB1*0301 allele was considerably higher in patients with endometriosis, relative to the controls. No appreciable difference was observed between the frequencies of DPB1 alleles between the patients and controls. The study projected possible implication of the HLA systems in the etiology of endometriosis; however, they recommended further study (Keisuke et al., 2002).

An in-depth study is warranted to identify HLA status in patients with and without endometriosis. It may possibly aid indiscriminating those with *proclivity* for endometriosis from normal persons. This may be used to implement preventive measures. Successful detection if any of HLA status of different racial/ethnic groups of patients with endometriosis may be of much epidemiological significance. Furthermore it may help counseling women about their risk of developing endometriosis.

The precise mechanism underlies action of dioxin and its similes (TCDD/PCBs) modifying the endometrial physiology still remains undefined. Besides it is conjecturably reason of the problem of evaluating the intrauterine exposure, childhood and adulthood in addition its real outcomes compounded by the constraints of its in vitro reliability. Thus it warrants further study to comprehend the mechanism of impact of these ecological pollutants, on reproductive health in particular, and general health of persons. Prevention tactics must include establishment of exposure limits. The plan must also investigate into procedures to diminish pollution and enhance use of our natural resources (Bellelis et al., 2011).

Subsequent to this study that reported that HLA-DRB1 alleles are described to be linked with the hazard of endometriosis in Japanese populations (Hee et al., 2006). Whang et al 2005 (b) conducted a study to verify whether vulnerability to advanced endometriosis is also related to HLA-DRB1 alleles in a Korean population, which is ethnically close to Japanese. Whang et al., 2005 did not find any association between predispositions of advanced endometriosis with HLA-DRB1 alleles in a Korean population, contrary to the case in the Japanese population.

This dissimilarity per se between two groups of researchers prompts further studies in different racial and other ethnic populations in various countries including Malaysia. It will also serve as an indicator for susceptibility to endometriosis. Large scale studies encompassing all the races and ethnic groups in Malaysia as well as in South East Asia are essential.

Alternative Medicine and Futuristic Projections:

From a limited review of the literature on ayurveda, it has become clear that this entity (endometriosis) is well recognized. However, the diagnosis and treatment of this condition is based on the constitution of the patient. Their holistic approach includes study of the pathology of the condition and management of these patients not only by therapeutic approach but also by regulation of diet and improvement of physical and mental status of the patient. Ayurvedic perception of pathology is that it is due to 'kapha' that generates surplus endometrial cells leading to the extra uterine transmission of cells. This system also recognizes the autoimmune nature of endometriosis which is in keeping with allopathic concept. It seems, to the best of my knowledge that the herbal therapy which is in use has not been systematically analyzed or confirmed. (Vaidya Atreya Smith –book on Ayurvedic Healing for Women)

The common use of Japanese herbal medicines (Kampo medicines) ranks as the third most favored therapeutic option for treatment of endometriosis in Japan. This old-fashioned therapy is meant for improving different signs and symptoms of endometriosis without lowering serum estradiol levels or producing menstrual disturbances (Tanaka 2000).

A coordinated collaborative research between practitioners of different systems of medicine such as Allopathy, Indian (Ayurveda), Japanese medicine, Korean medicine and Homeopathy is to be planned in involving large scale studies of different races with long term monitoring. It is essential to systematically analyse all the herbal extracts used by different systems. The active ingredient from these extracts have to be identified before testing its efficacy .It is equally important to test this ingredient in animals before recommending for human use.

Diagnosis of Endometriosis; Proteomics:

Before we deal with advances in proteomics a brief

discussion of the role of cytokines and their value in comprehending the exact pathogenesis of endometriosis and development of novel therapeutic strategies is merits mention. Systematic and extensive studies by computer search showed that the peritoneal fluid of women with endometriosis has an augmented population of activated macrophages which release growth factors and cytokines. Several cytokines were found to be raised in the peritoneal fluid of women with endometriosis. As the peritoneal milieu environment may be regulated by local factors, cytokines are alleged to have played a participatory role in the pathogenesis and evolution of endometriosis and endometriosis-related infertility. A possible pathogenic mechanism links cytokines with endometriosis (Harada et al., 2001). While elevated levels of several cytokines including interleukin (IL)-1, 6, 8, 10, tumor necrosis factor (TNF)-alpha, and vascular endothelial growth factor (VEGF) were found in the peritoneal fluid (PF) of women with endometriosis, there was decreased expression of some cytokines such as IL-2, and interferon (IFN)-gamma. The former cytokines may be implicated in macrophage activation, inflammatory change and increased angiogenesis, the latter cytokines mirror the lessened T- and natural killer (NK)-cell function. It is notable that endometriotic implants generate some factors, such as matrix metalloproteinases (MMPs), Bcl-2, and disturb their ability to implant into the peritoneum. Peritoneal cytokines, which are secreted by mesothelial cells, leukocytes and ectopic endometrial cells, interact locally and systemically in women with endometriosis (Wu and Ho 2003). Cytokines, which are generated by many kinds of cells including endometriotic tissues, have various roles in the pathogenesis of endometriosis and endometriosis-related infertility. Further research is warranted to determine the precise role of these cells and soluble factors that are required not only to enhance comprehension of endometriosis but also to develop new therapeutic strategies (Abrao et al., 1997). Additional research is mandatory for elucidating the precise role and relationships of these cytokines and this may be useful to shed light on .the comprehension of endometriosis and may be helpful to improve current therapies and provide new therapeutic approaches (May et al., 2010).

CA125 the cell surface antigen is expressed by offshoots of coelomic and mullerian epithelia it is regarded as the most frequent marker for diagnosis of endometriosis (Akita et al., 2012). Elevated levels of CA125t are found in the late phase of endometriosis the low sensitivity of CA125 renders its use limited in identification of early stage or mild endometriosis (Kitawaki et al 2005). Thus it is of little value for routine screening. It is well established that CA125 antigen also known as MUC16 is a helpful indicator for ovarian malignancy, but it is also found raised in endometriosis. Assessment of the sTn/MUC16 level is possibly valuable in differentiating endometriosis from ovarian malignancy; additionally it can be of useful for determining the clinical stage, cytological grade, and histological type of ovarian malignancy (Feeley et al 2001). Kitawaki et al. showed that the lack of precision of CA125 assay obviously promotes the need for transvaginal ultrasonography for early screening of endometriosis (Bischof et al., 1986).

As a prelude to the description of recent research advances some of the following biomarkers for endometriosis will be recapitulated for academic satisfactoriness:

CA125 in endometriosis:

CA125 is expressed as a membrane-bound protein at the surface of cells that undergo metaplastic differentiation into a Müllerian-type epithelium (Kenemans et al 1993; Tamakoshi et al., 1995). A widely studied biomarker CA125 has potential for use in the early detection of ovarian carcinoma (OC), and it has shown valuable in both detection and disease monitoring (Norum et al., 2001; Meden et al., 1998). Year ,many studies have reported raised levels of soluble CA125 in many other malignant conditions –as for instance breast cancer, (Ismail et al., 1994) gastric cancer (Bergan et al.,

2007),. CA125 levels have also been found elevated in benign conditions [such as endometriosis (Nathalie et al 2007). CA125 symbolizes a striking therapeutic target and several studies have been developing various strategies, including antibodies against CA125, anti-idiotype antibodies, antibodies specific for the membrane-bound form of CA125, and antibodies bound to cytotoxic drugs or fused with cytokines such as IL6. There is immense prospect for investigating all these approaches and should be dynamically pursued, especially in view of the dismal prognosis of OC (28). Various reports imply that CA125 precludes the fetal immunological rejection via its communications with NK cells, and the immune-evasive properties of ovarian carcinoma cells. Comprehending the CA-125 -provoked immunosuppressive tactics could be used to explore new therapies for autoimmune diseases including endometriosis and inflammatory disorders (Cho et al 2015).

C-reactive protein (CRP) is an acute phase protein and an inflammatory marker that is a prospective non-invasive biomarker of endometriosis. Its generation is stirred by pro-inflammatory cytokines such as IL-6, IL-1 and TNF-alpha (Jia et al 2015) which are up-regulated in women with endometriosis in comparison with controls (Rekker et al., 2015).

CRP is generally acknowledged as a biochemical marker of systemic inflammation and usually used in clinical setting as an indicator of infection, inflammation or tissue injury (Ledue et al 2001). Furthermore slightly increased CRP levels may signify a systemic subclinical inflammation in patients vulnerable to develop metabolic syndrome, colon cancer and cardiovascular disease (Abrao et al 1997)

A study by Abrao et al., 1997 evaluated CA 125 II, C-reactive protein (CRP) and serum amyloid A (SAA) and anticardiolipin antibody (aCL) levels for the diagnosis of pelvic endometriosis.. The study revealed that these determinations may help in the diagnosis and the indication of treatment for pelvic endometriosis. Both CA

125 II and CRP levels were elevated in advanced stages of compared with healthy controls, mainly during the first 3 days of the menstrual cycle; Calculation of CA 125 II concentrations at the onset of the menstrual cycle may assist the diagnosis of stage III and IV endometriosis. Apparently IgMaCL is linked with the occurrence of all stages of the disease, and SAA values are increased in severe states. Hence estimation of these molecules may be helpful in the diagnosis and management of endometriosis.

Conventional automated techniques for estimation of CRP characteristically have restricted sensitivity in the low range of CRP concentrations in peripheral blood (D'Hooghe et al 2006). A number of high sensitivity (hsCRP) assays have been established with enhanced sensitivity and accuracy at low concentrations of CRP with the object of determine subclinical inflammation (Roberts et al., 2001). Undeniably, needless to emphasise that high sensitivity of the assay may be of paramount value to ascertain low grade inflammation in plasma. Hence, the test to confirm the assumption that in plasma a high sensitivity CRP assay (hsCRP assay) is more precise than a classical CRP assay (classical CRP) to ascertain low grade inflammation in plasma of women with endometriosis. This study (Roberts et al., 2001), confirmed the superiority of hsCRP assay over the traditional CRP assay for the determination of subclinical inflammation in plasma of endometriosis patients. The findings of this study were in keeping with the observations of other researchers (Poddubnyy et al 2010). These studies found elevated levels of hsCRP but not CRP levels, in sera from patients. There was a closer link between hsCRP levels with the advanced stage of disease compared to CRP levels (Poddubnyy et al 2010; Kalsch et al 2010).

A brief reference to antiendometrial antibodies is relevant here.

The changes in humoral and cell-mediated immunity subscribe to the endometriosis-related female infertility

(Vassiliadis et al., 2005). Furthermore, endometriosis has been regarded as an autoimmune disorder associated with other autoimmune diseases.. Conventional autoimmune diseases, including endometriosis, are typified by polyclonal B-cell activation and generation of many diverse autoantibodies [Gleicher et al., 1987]. Approximately 40%–60% of patients with endometriosis exhibit increased autoantibody response to a panel of autoantigens (Lebovic et al 2001). They frequently comprise specific antiendometrial antibodies (Sarapik et al 2010;, Lang et al 2001; Mathur, 1999), but also antiovarian antibodies AOA, antinuclear autoantibodies (ANA), smooth muscle autoantibodies (SMA), and antiphospholipid antibodies (APA) (Geva et al., 1997; Mathur et al., 1982; Ulcová-Gallová et al., 2002)

Nisenblatet al., 2016 who included in their141 studies involving 15,141 participants assessed 122 blood biomarkers. All the studies including anti endometrial antibodies were deprived of methodological quality. In 4 studies involving 759 women revealed mean sensitivities and specificities of anti-endometrial antibodies were 0.81 (95% confidence interval (CI) 0.76 to 0.87) and 0.75 (95% CI 0.46 to 1.00).

Sera from 42 patients with infertility were assessed by indirect immunofluorescence for the occurrence of antiendometrial antibodies. While 24 out of 28 patients with positive antibody had endometriosis, there was no association between the grade of immunofluorescence and the clinical rigor of endometriosis. It is proposed that this has the potential to be used as a noninvasive immunological test for endometriosis (Robert and Charles 1985).

A brief consideration of miRNAS in endometriosis is aimed at highlighting the recent strides in research based on state of the art technologies .recent research has illustrated the role of miRNAs in the pathogenesis of endometriosis .miRNAsare strong controllers of gene expression in all vital processes- including cell survival, matrix remodeling cellular proliferation and angiogneisis implicated in the origin and development of endometriosis (Josep et al., 2016 ; Laudanski et al., 2015).

Exploration of circulating miRNAs as bioindicators of endometriosis is an evolving arena of research, and thus far just a few studies have reported both in serum (Cho et al., 2015) and plasma (Jia et al., 2013; Rekker et al., 2015). Evaluation of expression of three miRNAs (miR-200a-3p, miR-200b-3p, and miR-141-3p) in plasma of 61 patients and 65 control women revealed ddown regulation of all three miRNAs in patients and miR-200a-3p and miR-141-3p displayed the maximum potential as noninvasive biomarkers for endometriosis. Notably, differences in the levels of the three miRNAs were noticed with lower levels in evening samples, possibly because of daily vacillations in their expression.

Although reports of differences in mRNA expression between endometriotic lesions and eutopic endometrium from women with endometriosis have appeared in the literature (Ohlsson et al., 2009). Limited studies have concentrated on variances between eutopic endometrium from women with and without endometriosis study (Ohlsson et al., 2009).

Burney et al. analysed the miRNA expression profile in the endometrium of women with and without endometriosis .Burney et al using miRNA arrays with subsequent qRT-PCR confirmation described downregulation of four miRNAs (miR-34c-5p, miR-9, miR-9*, miR-34b*) in the eutopic endometrium from women with endometriosis in comparison with control endometrium. Study (Laudanski et al. 2015). Brief consideration of miRNAs in endometriosis is aimed at highlighting the recent strides in research based on state of the art technologies.Recent research has illustrated the role of miRNAs in the pathogenesis of endometriosis .miRNAs are strong controllers of gene expression in all vital processes- including cell survival, matrix remodeling cellular proliferation and angiogneisis implicated in the origin and development of endometriosis (Hughes et al., 1993).

Exploration of circulating miRNAs as bioindicators of endometriosis is an evolving arena of research, and thus far just a few studies have reported both in and plasma serum (Cho et al 2015). Evaluation of expression of three miRNAs (miR-200a-3p, miR-200b-3p, and miR-141-3p) in plasma of 61 patients and 65 control women revealed down regulation of all three miRNAs in patients and miR-200a-3p and miR-141-3p displayed the maximum potential as noninvasive biomarkers for endometriosis. Notably, differences in the levels of the three miRNAs were noticed with lower levels in evening samples, possibly because of daily vacillations in their expression.

Although reports of differences in miRNA expression between endometriotic lesions and eutopic endometrium from women with endometriosis have appeared in the literature (Braza-Boïls et al., 2016). Limited studies have concentrated on variances between eutopic endometrium from women with and without endometriosis (Braza-Boïls et al., 2016).

Burney et al. analysed the miRNA expression profile in the endometrium of women with and without endometriosis (Burney et al 2009). Burney et al using miRNA arrays with subsequent qRT-PCR confirmation described downregulation of four miRNAs (miR-34c-5p, miR-9, miR-9 *, miR-34b *) in the eutopic endometrium from women with endometriosis in comparison with control endometrium study. Laudanski et al. of 25 women without endometriosis and 21 cases of ovarian endometriosis in which the expression of 667 human miRNAs was tested using PCR arrays confirmed the downregulation of miR-483-5p, , and miR-629-3p, in the eutopic endometrium of patients relative to controls. Exploration of circulating miRNAs as bioindicators of endometriosis is an evolving arena of research, and thus far just a few studies have reported both in serum and plasma. Evaluation of expression of three miRNAs (miR-200a-3p, miR-200b-3p, and miR-141-3p) in plasma of 61 patients and 65 control women revealed that all three miRNAs were downregulated in patients and miR-200a-

3p and miR-141-3p displayed the utmost potential as noninvasive biomarkers for endometriosis. Notably, differences of the levels of the three miRNAs were noticed. In this context the observations of Ohlsson Teague et al (2009) merit mention. By means of Microarray analysis it was possible to identify miRNA expression in matching ectopic and eutopic endometrial tissues equal to 14 up-regulated (miR-145, miR-143, miR-99a, miR-99b, miR-126, miR-100, miR-125b, miR-150, miR-125a, miR-223, miR-194, miR-365, miR-29c and miR-1) and eight down-regulated (miR-200a, miR-141, miR-200b, miR-142-3p, miR-424, miR-34c, miR-20a and miR-196b) miRNAs. Quantitative RT-PCR ratified disparity in expression of six miRNAs. In silico analysis recognized 3851 mRNA transcripts as hypothetical targets of the 22 miRNAs. , Of these microarray analysis revealed 673 miRNAS were differentially expressed in ectopic opposed to eutopic endometrial tissue. Functional analysis signified that the 673 miRNA targets comprise molecular pathways linked to endometriosis, together with c-Jun, CREB-binding protein, protein kinase B (Akt), and cyclin D1 (CCND1) signaling. Apparently these pathways are synchronized both transcriptionally as well as by miRNAs at posttranscriptional level. This study implied that the 22 miRNAs and their related mRNA target series symbolize pathways that support endometriosis. In view of that, miRNAs are prospective therapeutic targets for the treatment of endometriosis of 25 women without endometriosis and 21 cases of ovarian endometriosis in which the expression of 667 human miRNAs was tested using PCR arrays confirmed the downregulation of miR-483-5p, , and miR-629-3p, in the eutopic endometrium of patients relative to controls 27. Exploration of circulating miRNAs as bioindicators of endometriosis is an evolving arena of research, and thus far just a few studies have reported both in serum and plasma (Cho et al., 2015).. Evaluation of expression of three miRNAs (miR-200a-3p, miR-200b-3p, and miR-141-3p) in plasma of 61 patients and 65 control women revealed that all three miRNAs were downregulated in patients and miR-200a-3p and miR-141-3p displayed the utmost potential as noninvasive biomarkers for endometriosis. Notably, differences of the levels of the three miRNAs were noticed .Lower levels were found in evening samples, possibly because of daily oscillations in their expression. This denotes the significance of the time of collection as an essential factor to be considered while conducting circulating miRNAs studies.

While proteomics methods have been used to recognize proteins that would have the diagnostic potential as biomarkers of endometriosis, until 2012 most studies have been beset with difficulty in selecting and fractionating pertinent low-abundance proteins from myriads of proteins in the blood. The chief problems to be resolved are the selection of sample for recognizing new biomarkers and the categorization of test samples. The application of state of the art innovative technologies including fractionation techniques should help resolve this problem; amalgamation of novel non-gel-based proteomic procedures and different protein labeling approaches coupled with the current expansion of sophisticated bio-informatics implements have to achieve success in the discovery of comparatively non-invasive diagnostic tests for endometriosis.

Zhoa et al., 2015 had tested earlier the suitability of 2-DE gels and peptide mass mapping to identify candidate endometrial proteins by surface-enhanced laser desorption/ionization time-of-flight mass spectrometry (SELDI-TOF-MS) protein chip array technology, to detect proteomic patterns in serum of women with EM. However, The extremely low reproducibility and inability to detect low-abundance proteins has disapproved the use of SELDI technology. The ClinProt system facilitates preparation and acquisition of complex proteomic profile patterns and their comparative analyses. It can optimize searches for biomarkers. In the study, we used ClinProt technology to explore and identify biomarkers from serum of EM patients. Proteins which rendered identifying these proteins difficult.

According to an earlier study, expression of the ATP synthase β subunit ATP1B4 differed between patients with endometriosis and normal controls. This implies a possible link between ATP function and origin and evolution of endometriosis ClinProt identification of biomarkers for EM screening shows that it is decisive even for early-stage or minimal EM. Zhao et al (2015) detected five stable peaks with molecular weights of 4210, 5264, 2660, 5635, and 5904 Da as probable EM bioindicators. The link between ATP1B4 and FGA and EM pathogenesis warrants further study.

Advances in Proteomics research is further confirmed by many others including Fowler et al 2007. Despite the varied nature of endometrium, their study detected an array of dysregulated proteins in women with endometriosis which comprised: (i) molecular chaperones including heat shock protein 90 and annexin A2, (ii) proteins implicated in cellular redox state, such as peroxiredoxin 2, (iii) proteins involved in protein and DNA formation/breakdown, including ribonucleoside-diphosphatereductase, prohibitin and prolyl 4-hydroxylase(iv) secreted proteins, such as apolipoprotein A1

Functions of these proteins point toward their possible role in the pathogenesis of endometriosis. Moreover the studyconfirmed that 2-DE gel analysis and mass spectroscopic protein identification are appropriate for the recognition of proteins with candidate links with endometriosis. They recommended the utilization of these techniques on a greater scale to discover novel endometriosis-linked proteins, thus enhancing the comprehension of this multifaceted disease. A brief consideration of infertility and endometriosis is pertinent at this juncture. The relationship between endometriosis and infertility has been a hotly disputed subject for many years.

Administration of TNF binding proteins to block TNF alpha activity, simultaneously as one introduces menstrual endometrium, then one can substantially impede the development of endometriosis in baboons. Moreover, it is entirely possible to prevent the development of endometriosis-related adhesions.(Hooghe). Recent advances in the comprehensionof pathophysiology of endometriosis, have favored the perception of endometriosis an autoimmune disorder. Thus novel therapies using immunomodulators and other novel compounds are recommended. An ideal drug would be one that treats endometriosis without hampering fertility.

A study was performed to test the link between frequency of creative productivity and stage of endometriosis in keeping with their management. The study enrolled 151 consecutive women with laparoscopically confirmed endometriosis stage-1 and 2. Of these 49 cases underwent operative laparoscopy, 59 received medical therapy and 43 cases had undergone expectant management. During a two year duration the collective pregnancy rates were observed to be 36.7%, 30.5% and 20.9% respectively. The likelihood of continuing pregnancy further than 20 weeks were 30.6%, 25.4% and 16.2% correspondingly 21. The productivity of normal couples, was in the range of 0.15 to 0.20 per month and declines as age advances (Schwartz and Mayaux 1982; Hughes et al., 1995). In addition, endometriosis is associated with a lesser frequency of live birth (Collins et al., 1995).

At this juncture it is worth mentioning endometriosis is associated with Infertility and women with infertility have 6 to 8 folds more prone to develop endometriosis than fertile women (Verkauf 1987).

In spite of comprehensive research, there has been lack of unanimity of agreement and consequently several mechanisms have been postulated to elucidate the link between endometriosis and infertility. These mechanisms comprise abnormal pelvic anatomy, endocrine aberrations and changes in peritoneal function, as well as hormonal and cell-mediated functions in the endometrium.

Current emphasis is on large scale multicentre studies, which should include controls. Interdisciplinary and multidisciplinary approach augurs well to enhance understanding of the pathogenesis and other aspects of endometriosis, which remain to be clearly defined.

International collaboration with centers of excellence will contribute considerably to fine tune research. From research point of view, it has become amply clear that there is a paradigm shift from the conventional hypothesis driven research to evidence based and patient centric research. The value of hypothesis driven research is no doubt indisputable but in modern era, is in favor favoring which emphasizes evidence based medicine and thus this justifies evidence based medicine research. Successful implementation suggested recommendations with resultant promising results will undoubtedly and meaningfully add a robust fiber to the magnificent fabric of research in endometriosis.

References

Abrao MS; Podgaec S; Filho BM; Ramos LO; Pinotti JA. and de Oliveira RM (1997). The use of biochemical markers in the diagnosis of pelvic endometriosis. Hum Reprod. 12(11); 2523-2527.

Akita K; Yoshida S; Ikehara Y; Shirakawa S; Toda M;

Inoue M; Kitawaki J; Nakanishi H; Narimatsu H. and Nakada H. (2012). Different levels of sialyl-Tn antigen expressed on MUC16 in patients with endometriosis and ovarian cancer. Int J Gynecol Cancer. 22(4); 531-538.

Bellelis, P, Podgaec, S. and Abrão, M. S. (2011). Environmental factors and endometriosis.Rev Assoc Med Bras (1992). 57(4); 448-452.

Bergan L, Gross JA, Nevin B, Urban N, Scholler N (2007). Development and in vitro validation of anti-mesothelinbiobodies that prevent CA125/Mesothelin-dependent cell attachment. Cancer Lett.

Bischof P, Tseng L, Brioschi PA, Herrmann WL (1986). Cancer antigen 125 is produced by human endometrial stromal cells. Hum Reprod. ;1:423-426.

Braza-Boïls A., Marí-Alexandre J., Gilabert J., Sánchez-Izquierdo D., España F., Estellés A., Gilabert-Estellés J. MicroRNA expression profile in endometriosis: Its relation to angiogenesis and fibrinolytic factors. Hum. Reprod. 2014;29:978-988.

Cho S; Mutlu L; Grechukhina O and Taylor H. S. (2015). Circulating microRNAs as potential biomarkers for endometriosis. Fertil Steril. 103(5); 1252-1260.

Collins JA, Burrows EA, Wilan AR (1995). The prognosis for live birth among untreated infertile couples. Fertil Steril.;64(1):22-28.

D'Hooghe TM, Kyama C, Debrock S, Meuleman C, and Mwenda JM (2004). Future directions in endometriosis research.Ann N Y Acad Sci. 1034:316-325.

Dong Hee; Whang Sung; Hoon Kim; Young Min; Choi

Myoung; Hee ParkJi; Hyun Noh and Yong Bong Kim (2006). No association between HLA-DRB1 alleles and susceptibility to advanced stage endometriosis in a Korean population Human Reproduction. Volume 21, Issue 1, Pages 129-133.

Endometriosis: current and future medical therapiesBest Practice & Research Clinical Obstetrics & Gynaecology. Volume 22, Issue 2.

Feeley KM, Wells M (2001). Precursor lesions of ovarian epithelial malignancy. Histopathology. ;38:87-95.

Forges T, Monnier-Barbarino P, Faure GC, Béné MC. Autoimmunity and antigenic targets in ovarian pathology. Human Reproduction Update. 2004;10(2):163-175.

Geva E, Amit A, Lerner-Geva L, Lessing JB (1997). Autoimmunity and reproduction. Fertility and Sterility.;67(4):599-611.

Gleicher N, El-Roeiy A, Confino E, Friberg J (1987). Is endometriosis an autoimmune disease? Obstetrics & Gynecology. ;70(1):115-122.

Harada T; Iwabe T. and Terakawa N. (2001). Role of cytokines in endometriosis. Fertil Steril. 76(1); 1-10.

Harmeet Malhotra (2009). Senior Consultant, Department of Obstetrics & Gynaecology, Indraprastha Apollo Hospitals, Sarita Vihar, New Delhi 110 076, India

Hughes EG, Fedorkow DM, Cllins JA (1993). A quantitative overview of controlled trials in endometriosis-associated infertility. Fertil Steril.;59:963-970.

Ismail MA, Rotmensch J, Mercer LJ, Block BS, Salti GI, Holt JA (1994). CA-125 in peritoneal fluid from patients with nonmalignant gynecologic disorders. J Reprod Med.;39:510-512.

Jia S.Z.; Yang Y.; Lang J.; Sun P., and Leng J. (2013). Plasma miR-17-5p, miR-20a and miR-22 are down-regulated in women with endometriosis. Hum. Reprod. 28; 322-330.

Kalsch AI, Csernok E, Munch D, Birck R, Yard BA, Gross W, Kalsch T, Schmitt WH (2010). Use of Highly Sensitive C-Reactive Protein for Followup of Wegener's Granulomatosis. Journal of Rheumatology.;37:2319-2325.

Keisuke Ishii; Koichi Takakuwa; Takuya Mitsui and Kenichi Tanaka (2002). Studies on the human leukocyte antigen-DR in patients with endometriosis: genotyping of HLA-DRB1 alleles Human Reproduction. Volume 17, Issue 3, Pages 560-582.

Kenemans P, Yedema CA, Bon GG, von Mensdorff-Pouilly S. (1993). CA 125 in gynecological pathology--a review. Eur J ObstetGynecolReprod Biol.;49:115-124.

Kitawaki J; Ishihara H; Koshiba H; Kiyomizu M; Teramoto M. and Kitaoka Y. (2005). Usefulness and limits of CA-125 in diagnosis of endometriosis without associated ovarian endometriomas. Hum Reprod. 20(2 Suppl1);1999-2003.

Lang GA, Yeaman GR (2001). Autoantibodies in endometriosis sera recognize a Thomsen-Friedenreich-like carbohydrate antigen. Journal of Autoimmunity.;16(2):151-161.

Lebovic DI, Mueller MD (2001)., Taylor RN. Immunobiology of endometriosis. Fertility and Sterility.;75(1):1-10.

Ledue TB, Rifai N (2001). High sensitivity immunoassays

for C-reactive protein: Promises and pitfalls. Clin Chem Lab Med.;39:1171-1176.

Mathur S, Peress MR, Williamson HO (1982). Autoimmunity to endometrium and ovary in endometriosis. Clinical and Experimental Immunology. ;50(2):259-266.

Mathur SP, Lee JH, Jiang H, Arnaud P, Rust PF (1999). Levels of transferrin and alpha 2-HS glycoprotein in women with and without endometriosis. Autoimmunity.;29(2):121-127.

May K.E; S.A Conduit-Hulbert J; Villar S.; Kirtley S.H. and Kennedy C.M. (2010). Becker Peripheral biomarkers of endometriosis: a systematic review Human Reproduction Update, Volume 16, Issue 6, Pages 651-674.

Meden H, Fattahi-Meibodi A (1999).. CA 125 in benign gynecological conditions. Int J Biol Markers. 1998;13:231-237.

Nathalie Scholler 1 and Nicole Urban2 CA125 in Ovarian CancerBiomark Med. 2007 Dec; 1(4): 513-523.doi: 10.2217/17520363.1.4.513

New Developments in Medical Management of Endometriosis Apollo Medicine. Volume 6, Issue 3; Pages 247-255.

Nisenblat V1, Bossuyt PM, Shaikh R, Farquhar C, Jordan V, Scheffers CS, Mol BW, Johnson N, Hull ML.Blood biomarkers for the non-invasive diagnosis of endometriosis.Cochrane Database Syst Rev. 2016 May 1;(5):CD012179.

Norum LF, Erikstein B, Nustad K. Elevated CA125 in breast cancer--A sign of advanced disease. Tumour Biol. 2001;22:223-228.

Paolo Vercellini, (2008). Edgardo Somigliana, MD, PhD

(Clinical Assistant)

Paul A. Fowler, Jenny Tattum, Siladitya Bhattacharya, Thomas Klonisch, Sabine Hombach-Klonisch, RafetGazvani, Richard G. Lea, Iain Miller, William G. Simpson and Phillip Cash (2007). An investigation of the effects of endometriosis on the proteome of hum Proteomics. 7; 130–142.

Poddubnyy DA, Rudwaleit M, Listing J, Braun J, Sieper J (2010). Comparison of a high sensitivity and standard C reactive protein measurement in patients with ankylosing spondylitis and non-radiographic axial spondyloarthritis. Annals of the Rheumatic Diseases.;69:1338–1341.

Rasheed K, Atta H, TF Taha, O Azmy, D Sabry, M Selim, A El-Sawaf, M Bibars, A Ramzy, W El-Garf, and M Anwar (2010). A Novel Endometriosis Inducing Factor. In Women with EndometriosisJ Stem Cells Regen Med.; 6(3): 157–164.

Rekker K.; Saare M.; Roost A. M.; Kaart T.; Sõritsa D.; Karro H.; Sõritsa A.; Simón C.; Salumets A. and Peters M. (2015). Circulating miR-200-family micro-RNAs have altered plasma levels in patients with endometriosis and vary with blood collection time. Fertil. Steril. 104; 938–946.

Richard, O. Burney, M.D. and Linda C. Giudice, (2012). Pathogenesis and Pathophysiology of EndometriosisFertilSteril. 98(3): 1010-1016.

Robert Allen Wild Md Charles Alex Shivers (1985), Antiendometrial Antibodies in Patients With EndometriosisAmerican journal ofReproductive Immunology July1985.

Rogers, PA, D'Hooghe TM, Fazleabas A, Giudice LC, Montgomery GW, PetragliaF. and Taylor RN (2013). Defining future directions for endometriosis research: workshop report from the 2011 World

Congress of Endometriosis In Montpellier, France. Reprod Sci. 20(5): 483-499.

Sarapik A, Haller-Kikkatalo K, Utt M, Teesalu K, Salumets A, Uibo R. Serum anti-endometrial antibodies in infertile women—potential risk factor for implantation failure. American Journal of ReproductiveImmunology. 2010;63(5):349–357.

Schwartz D, Mayaux MJ (1982). Female fecundity as a function of age: results of artificial insemination in 2193 nulliparous women with azoospermic husbands. CECOS. N Engl J Med.;306(7):404–406.

Stephen Kennedy; Agneta Bergqvist; Charles Chapron; Thomas D'Hooghe; Gerard Dunselman; Robert Greb Lone and HummelshojAndrew (2005). PrenticeErtan Saridogan on behalf of the ESHRE Special Interest Group for Endometriosis and Endometrium Guideline Development Group Human Reproduction, Volume 20, Issue 10, Pages 2698–2704.

Tamakoshi K, Kikkawa F, Hasegawa N, et al (1995). Clinical value of a new serum tumor marker, CA125II, in gynecologic disease: comparison with CA125. GynecolObstet Invest. ;39:125–129.

Tanaka T; Umesaki N; Mizuno K. and Fujino Ogita S. (2000). Anti-endometrial IgM autoantibodies in endometriotic patients: a preliminary study. ClinExpObstet Gynecol. 27(2):133-137.

Ulcová-Gallová Z, Bouše V, Švábek L, Turek J, Rokyta Z (2002). Endometriosis in reproductive immunology. American Journal of Reproductive Immunology. ; 47(5):269–274.

Vassiliadis S, Relakis K, Papageorgiou A, Athanassakis I (2005);. Endometriosis and infertility: a multi-cytokine imbalance versus ovulation, fertilization and early embryo development. Clinical &

Developmental Immunology.;12(2):125-129.

Vassiliadis S, Relakis K, Papageorgiou A, Athanassakis I. (2005);1 Endometriosis and infertility: a multi-cytokine imbalance versus ovulation, fertilization and early embryo development. Clinical & Developmental Immunology. ;12(2):125-129.

Verkauf BS (1987). The incidence, symptoms, and signs of endometriosis in fertile and infertile women. J Fla Med Assoc.;74(9):671-675.

Wu, M. Y. and Ho, H. N (2003). The role of cytokines in endometriosis. Am J ReprodImmunol. 49(5); 285-296.

Yang Zhao, Ya-Nan Liu, Yi Li, Li Tian, Xue Ye, Heng Cui, and Xiao-Hong Chang (2015). Identification of Biomarkers for Endometriosis Using Clinical ProteomicsChin Med J (Engl). 128(4): 520-527.

ABOUT THE AUTHOR

Dr. Methil Kannan Kutty; FRCPath (London), FRCPA (Australia), presently is Professor of Pathology in Faculty of Medicine, Lincoln University College, Malaysia. He held Professor of Pathology in University Islam Malaysia, UKM Malaysia, International Medical University Malaysia, Sheffield college of Medicine, King Faisal University, Dammam, KSA and UiTM Malaysia. He is the author of SIX books and he has published more than 160 papers in peer reviewed journals.

Dr. Muhamed T. Osman; MBChB, MSc PAT, PhD PAT, presently, is Associate Professor and Head of Pathology in Faculty of Medicine and Defence Health, National Defence University of Malaysia. He was Consultant Pathologist and Clinical Lecturer at Teaching Laboratories/ Medical City of Baghdad, Iraq and Senior Lecturer of Pathology at UiTM Malaysia. He is the author of TEN books and has published more than 145 papers in peer reviewed journals.

www.ingramcontent.com/pod-product-compliance
Lightning Source LLC
Chambersburg PA
CBHW052310220526
45472CB00001B/61